IDIOMS OF DISTRESS

Idioms of Distress

Psychosomatic Disorders in
Medical and Imaginative Literature

By
Lilian R. Furst

STATE UNIVERSITY OF NEW YORK PRESS

Published by
State University of New York Press, Albany

For information, address State University of New York Press,
90 State Street, Suite 700, Albany, NY 12207

Production by Christine L. Hamel
Marketing by Anne Valentine

Library of Congress Cataloging in Publication Data

Furst, Lilian R.
   Idioms of distress : psychosomatic disorders in medical and imaginative
literature / Lilian R. Furst.
      p. cm.
   Includes bibliographical references and index.
   ISBN 0-7914-5557-2 (hbk.: alk. paper) — ISBN 0-7914-5558-0 (pbk.: alk. paper)
   1. Medicine, Psychosomatic. 2. Literature and mental illness. 3. Imagination
in literature. 4. Diseases in literature. I. Title.

RC49.F87 2002
616.08—dc21   2002017723

10 9 8 7 6 5 4 3 2 1

Wer Augen hat zu sehen and Ohren zu hören, überzeugt sich, dass die Sterblichen kein Geheimnis verbergen können. Wessen Lippen schweigen, der schwätzt mit den Fingerspitzen; aus allen Poren dringt ihm der Verrat. Und darum ist die Aufgabe, das verborgenste Seelische bewusst zu machen, sehr wohl lösbar.

He that has eyes to see and ears to hear may convince himself that no mortal can keep a secret. If his lips are silent, he chatters with his finger-tips; betrayal oozes out of him at every pore. And thus the task of making conscious the most hidden recesses of the mind is one which it is quite possible to accomplish.

—Freud, *Bruchstück einer Hysterie-Analyse* (*Dora*)

Contents

Preface

"It's all in your head"; "Isn't that what women are supposed to get?" These two responses to the word "psychosomatic" (incidentally, from well-educated individuals) are vivid illustrations of the uncertainties surrounding both the term and the concept. Neither formulation is wholly incorrect: the "head" (i.e., the mind) plays a cardinal role in psychosomatic disorders, and the gender ratio is weighted on the female side.[1] Yet each of these phrases is at best only partially valid; the one carries an undertone of dismissiveness, while the interrogatory form of the other indicates hesitancy.

Why are psychosomatic disorders so resistant to ready understanding? Their recalcitrant nature is due in part to their multivalence; chameleon-like, they can assume many different guises, appearing in every part of the body, although some, such as headaches and stomachaches, are more common than others. Also, they are hard to diagnose, for they do not yield signs of pathological changes in test results. They remain elusive, cryptic, posing a challenge to sufferers and physicians alike. And beyond their overt, often puzzling manifestations, psychosomatic disorders encompass a deeper problem in their close intertwining of psyche and soma, as their name suggests.

Yet the term itself is not a rarity. We apply it, with a wry smile, to a sudden headache, for instance, brought on by an annoying encounter that has rubbed us up the wrong way. By recognizing the headache as psychosomatic, we perceive it as a physical outcome of, that is, an outlet for, an emotional state. We know that it is not purely imaginary: it is real—we may take Tylenol or Advil or whatever pain medication we prefer. We do not immediately believe it to be a symptom of a grave pathological disturbance such as a brain tumor. But *how* are mind and body interacting? By what paths is the annoyance translated, converted into the headache or the stomachache or some other symptom? While recent advances in the medical sciences offer some answers by reference to neurotransmitters, a great deal still remains unexplained at the beginning of the twenty-first century.

For this reason, all snappy definitions tend to be unsatisfactory. I have chosen as my title one I consider workable, "idioms of distress," which is taken from the latest edition of the American Psychiatric Association's *Diagnostic and Statistical Manual* (*DSM-IV,* 1994). The phrase was coined to designate what are known in medical language as somatoform disorders— "somatoform" having in the past twenty years superseded "psychosomatic" in professional terminology, as I shall later explain. Such disorders are described as "culturally shaped idioms of distress" that express concerns about a broad range of personal and social problems (450). Carefully worded though this definition is, it still begs a number of questions, not least the scope of "idiom."

According to the *Oxford English Dictionary,* an idiom is a form of expression, a construction, often having a meaning other than its grammatical or logical one. In its character as a construct, it denotes something newly created to fit a particular purpose, occasion, or situation. In its departure from (transcendence of) its strictly grammatical or logical meaning, an idiom moves toward metaphor, a mode of speech that entails a figurative transference from one medium to another. The word is, therefore, particularly apposite to psychosomatic disorders in shifting the focus from the manifest symptom itself onto its implicit metaphoricity.

This metaphoricity is one major source of the elusiveness so characteristic of the psychosomatic. We have difficulty in understanding not merely the term itself but what it represents because a kind of disguise is ingrained into the very concept. Not only does it comprise "a broad range of personal and social problems," it lacks a circumscribed psychopathology. The absence of a readily recognizable psychopathology to account for patients' complaints, while itself indicative of the potential for a psychosomatic disorder, intensifies the problem of distinguishing such an illness from organic disease. Physicians tend to be perplexed by patients whose symptoms do not fit into established syndromes and frustrated at having to run a long series of tests in order to rule out the possibility of an underlying pathology.[2] On the other hand, precisely this openness to multilayered interpretation and, above all, to metaphoricity make psychosomatic disorders an inviting terrain for reading from a literary angle. For literary study delights in the very ambivalence and figuration that are suspect to medicine, which must aim for the maximum certainty. Some of the fundamental issues at play in psychosomatic disorders are addressed in the opening chapter, "Speaking Through the Body."

Among the wide spectrum of somatoform disorders (pain disorder, hypochondriasis, body dysmorphic disorder, etc.), I have opted to concentrate on conversion disorders, whose hallmark is the translation of the distress into a physical symptom or symptoms, that is, its projection into the body as paralysis, deafness, blindness, muteness, or such lesser symptoms as headaches, palpitations, or gastrointestinal disturbances. Conversion disorders are the most common and striking among the psychosomatic disorders; they occur in 2.2 percent of the population, account for 5–10 percent of psychiatric consultations in general hospitals, and as high as 25–30 percent in Veterans Administration hospitals.[3] Their function as a nonverbal means of communication endows them with a metaphoric charge.

My study reaches from the mid-nineteenth century to the 1990s. Its second chapter, "Swings of the Historical Pendulum," offers a brief overview of the vicissitudes of psychosomatics in the past two centuries. The modulations in the cultural shapes of idioms of distress over the course of time have been examined by Edward Shorter in *From Paralysis to Fatigue: A History of Psychosomatic Illness in the Modern Era*. Taking psychosomatic illness as "any illness in which physical symptoms, produced by the action of the unconscious mind, are defined by the individual as evidence of organic disease and for which medical help is sought" (x), Shorter catalogues its successive incarnations in a series of forms predominant at different periods: spinal irritation, disorders of the pelvic organs in women, motor disturbances (paralysis), dissociation (somnambulism and catalepsy), neurasthenia, pain, and chronic fatigue. His study illustrates, alongside the extraordinary range of psychosomatic manifestations, the varying and often bizarre theories about their physical manifestations. However, Shorter is concerned only with changing symptomatologies and belief systems without regard to their metaphoricity or psychological etiology, and he does not cover imaginative literature.

Shorter's book and other studies such as Janet Beizer's *Ventriloquized Bodies* raise an awkward terminological dilemma in their use of the word "hysteria." Commonly—and frequently rather loosely—it has been applied to the kinds of disorders subsequently deemed psychosomatic or nowadays somatoform. I prefer to use the more current terms for the sake of both greater precision and gender neutrality. As far as possible, I avoid "hysteria," since it carries pejorative connotations as well as considerable political baggage. Adopted enthusiastically in the cultural arena, it has quickly become hackneyed. Significantly, it has long been banished from psychiatric nosology because of its indeterminacy. I trace the evolution of psychiatric usage in the twentieth century in the third chapter, "The Mysterious Leap."

My primary focus is on the representation of psychosomatic disorders exhibited by fictional characters, not a biographical study of their authors' ills. If remote diagnosis in biography is a tricky enterprise, it is even more so in regard to fictional figures where the sole evidence consists of the author's words. This difficulty is discussed in the fourth chapter, "Literary Patients." From the available information I relate the protagonists' symptoms to today's criteria for psychosomatic disorders. At the same time I maintain an awareness, in relation to the earlier works, of the shifts in terminology, such as changes in the understanding of the term "nerves."

But rather than attempting to pin a precise diagnosis on a fictional figure, I am experimenting with a medical humanities methodology. Its foremost strength lies in its capacity for a multidimensional approach that envisages a complaint as much from a social and psychological perspective as from a biomedical angle. As Dr. Allen Barbour learned in his work at the Stanford Medical Center's Diagnostic Clinic, patients have to be seen not solely as bearers of syndromes but "as persons in family and social systems."[4] Such a comprehensive vision is vital in dealing with psychosomatic disorders where the customary medico-scientific model draws a blank. For the center of gravity of psychosomatics resides, as Zbigniew Lipowski has insisted, in the "interactional aspects of man's functioning."[5] The core of the psychosomatic disorder is at the interstices of mind and body, individual and environment, conscious and unconscious, distress and illness. To cite Helen Dunbar's pioneering work, *Emotions and Bodily Change*, "[T]he problem of psychosomatic interelationships is continually a stumbling-block to the [medical] specialist";[6] the royal road to better understanding necessitates attention to the wider psychodynamic factors that form the frame for and often the basis of the disorder itself.

One result of this realization is to assign cardinal importance to literary works in the endeavor to grasp the etiology of psychosomatic disorders. Through its generous breadth the literary text is the ideal forum in which to show the psychosocial constellations that impell individuals to speak through their bodies. The literary work opens up to analysis the cultural factors that provoke and shape idioms of distress. The complex amalgam of tensions and pressures, inter- and intrapersonal conflicts is available for probing as the impetus to the gradual crescendo of distress that is ultimately converted into a physical idiom.

My aim is, therefore, to engage in dualistic readings in which the partly speculative medicalized perception of an overt text of bodily disturbance is partnered by a humanistic perspective that interprets the literal as a metaphoric figuration of a psychological subtext. Such an approach capitalizes on the special aptitude of literary portrayals for showing the web of social entanglements and personal relationships in which the individual is embedded and entrapped. A contextualizing view of this kind can trace both the processes that promote the growth of a psychosomatic disorder as it evolves and those that foster its dissipation as healing sets in.

My choice of texts, though seemingly idiosyncratic, is governed by certain principles. There are ample instances of conversion disorders in nineteenth- and twentieth-century literature, but often they are no more than slight, transient indispositions, such as the headaches that Jane Austen's and Proust's protagonists suffer at moments of reversal and discouragement. Even a severe conversion such as the mutism of the eight-year-old Clara Hutch, who is struck dumb after witnessing her mother's shooting of her two brothers and attempt to kill her in Caleb Carr's *Angel of Darkness* (1997), may form just a small, episodic part of a work.

Sometimes doubt arises whether a character has an organic disease. Milly Theale in Henry James's *The Wings of the Dove* (1902) is a good example. Her consultations with the eminent physician Sir Luke Strett for an "unnamed woe" (299) are remarkably inconclusive. Does she have "a bad case of lungs . . . that [are] past patching," as some in her circle aver (265)? Many readers assume with Susan Sontag that Milly has tuberculosis.[7] Rita Charon, on the other hand, argues that Milly undergoes psychotherapy with Sir Luke.[8] A clearer but still murky case of conversion is Lise, the adolescent in Dostoyevsky's *Brothers Karamazov* (1880). At the beginning of the novel she is in a wheelchair, her legs paralyzed. Later she makes a spontaneous recovery. The circumstances remain mysterious, rooted perhaps in the tension between her and her mother, a widow still young and eager for suitors. That domineering, unstable mother may wish to forestall competition from her blooming, attractive daughter by infantilizing—and disabling—her. As Lise matures and wins the admiration of Alyosha, she gains the confidence to rise to her feet.

But such a reading is largely conjectural, and that is the crux of the difficulty in many of the literary portrayals of a conversion disorder. My criterion has been to seek out works where the evidence is sound, providing sufficient density of circumstantial detail as a cogent basis for interpretation. Such density, together with an extensive temporal stretch, makes it possible to follow the psychosocial hurts that lead to a conversion disorder as well as its end stage in the manifest symptom. So, although the works discussed are quite dissimilar, they all share a common feature, namely that the psychosomatic disorder is both well delineated and absolutely central to the entire plot. Their very diversity reveals the wide spectrum of culturally shaped idioms of distress.

It is a great pleasure to acknowledge the help given to me by so many friends and colleagues from various fields. Roger Spencer, M.D., provided me with a starter reading list of the important recent medical writing on psychosomatics. Mark Perlroth, M.D. recommended Barbour's *Caring for Patients,* and during my summers at Stanford not only lent a willing ear but also offered provocative responses. Stephen M. Ford, M.D., Tom Boeker, M.D., and C. Fred Irons, M.D., have listened with infinite patience to my lamentations about the difficulties of this project and have contributed constructive suggestions. I am grateful to Janice H. Koelb for the long-term loan of her *DSM-IV*, to Inger S. B. Brodey for drawing my attention to the *Synopsis of Psychiatry*, and to Peter Jacobson, M.D., for the loan of *Merritt's Textbook of Neurology*. Indeed, the entire Jacobson family—Peter, Karen, Kirstin, and Lars—has participated by suggesting works for inclusion. Diane McKenzie of the University of North Carolina's Health Sciences Library and Suzanne Porter of Duke University's Medical History Library have both given me valuable assistance. I am indebted to the University of North Carolina's Psychiatry and Literature reading group for introducing me to Flannery O'Connor's story "The Enduring Chill." My deepest gratitude goes to those who have bestowed on me the inestimable gift of encouragement: Joseph Frank, Edith Gelles, Steven and Madeline Levine, and, as ever, especially Esther Zago. A succession of graduate students have acted as my legs: S. Vida Grubisha, Gena Lewis, William A. Nolan, Thomas Spencer, and Marina Alexandrova; without their willing help this book could not have come into being.

PART I

Hiding and Seeking Distress

CHAPTER ONE

Speaking through the Body

Man has no Body distinct from his Soul.
—William Blake, *The Marriage*
of Heaven and Hell

In *Caring for Patients* Dr. Allen Barbour reports on a number of challenging cases that led him to a more successful method of treating them. Barbour headed the Diagnostic Clinic, part of the General Medical Clinic at Stanford University Medical Center, a tertiary care facility to which patients are referred when physicians elsewhere have not been able to diagnose and handle their complaints. Many of Barbour's patients had received medical attention for several years, had undergone all sorts of advanced tests and examinations, yet either showed no improvement or actually kept getting worse.

A typical case is that of Joseph H., a sixty-seven-year old widower, who complained of feeling "lightheaded, dizzy" for the eighteen months prior to admission. The patient had no other specific symptoms and an unremarkable medical history. He had shown no recognizable disease either at the routine physical examination and laboratory tests or at the elaborate workup, which included a comprehensive (and expensive) series of technological procedures to detect disease. Six or more potential syndromes, some quite rare, had been considered in the process of differential diagnosis. None fitted, nor had Joseph's dizziness yielded to therapeutic trials of various drugs such as antihistamines, anticoagulants, vasodilators, and antidepressants. By the time he was sent to Stanford, both he and his doctors were discouraged. However, to Barbour's own surprise, when he saw Joseph, "the source of his illness was clear from his initial response" (11). He quotes the patient's words, which revealed the crux of the problem: "Doctor, I feel dizzy nearly all the time since my wife died. I don't know what to do with myself. I'm confused. I watch TV, but I'm not interested. I go outside, but there's no place to go" (11). Recently moved to California, with no children, close friends, or special interests, he expressed his confusion as, and in, "dizziness." Joseph is a fine example of speaking through the body. Barbour comments: "He was a lonely man who had not yet assimilated his grief or learned to develop a new life. His personal situation *was* the clinical problem, and the key to its solution" (11). The remedy for Joseph's dizziness lay not in a medication but in being persuaded by a social worker to join a club where he could share activities.

Barbour chronicles many similar instances where he was able to remove or alleviate puzzling symptoms that had previously defied diagnosis. Jean G., a fifty-five-year old homemaker with three grown-up children who visited often, appeared to have no problems to account for the debilitating headaches that had become increasingly severe in the past three years. They were so intense that she was taking unusually high daily doses of codeine and visiting the emergency room about twice a month for injections of Demerol. Her marriage was loving and communicative; the couple had a nice home and no economic worries or concerns about their sexual relationship. Barbour decided "to view Jean in terms of her social situation. . . . I asked, 'What do you do?' 'Housework.' Then what? Long silence. So I asked, 'What else?' 'More housework'" (74). Barbour realized that, with her children married and successfully launched in their careers, "Jean had run out of purpose" (74); her life was barren for lack of meaningful social, athletic, intellectual, artistic, or recreational interests of significance to her. Encouraged to develop a minor hobby into an active business, making and selling greetings cards, Jean was able to dispense with the heavy drugs and to manage her occasional headaches with over-the-counter analgesics.

With Joseph and Jean, Barbour's nonmedical intervention resulted in changes in their lives that made a positive difference and so paved the way for improvement in their health. Even when no immediate, decisive modification ensues, a patient may be helped through understanding the underlying roots of the current symptomatology. This is what happened with Ruth B., a twenty-one-year old married dental assistant with one child who had had persistent pelvic pain in the right lower quadrant of her abdomen, plus occasional vomiting and constipation, irregular periods, and headaches. Over nineteen months she had been seen by sixteen physicians on twenty outpatient visits, four of them to the emergency room; she had been hospitalized three times, and, after X rays and other studies produced normal results, she had undergone an exploratory laparotomy with an appendectomy. Her doctors had recorded twenty possible diagnoses and tried four drug treatments. Her pelvic pains were ascribed to "obscure cause" (16) and compartmentalized, that is, never connected to her headaches. It was finally a student physician, "kindly, accepting, open-minded" (16), who had the insight that Ruth was suffering "from an emotional illness expressed as pelvic pain" (16). Without difficulty he elicited her story of material and sexual anxieties, which she readily opened up.

Another patient, Orvieta T., was, like Ruth, helped by being enabled to grasp the source of her symptomatology, despite the fact that there seemed to be no prospect of her breaking out of the vicious circle in which she was trapped. A sixty-two-year old married woman, Orvieta had, besides well-controlled asthma, persistent abdominal pains, headaches, backaches, and joint and muscle pains. She brought to the Diagnostic Clinic several pounds of X rays and results of assorted tests carried out over the previous three years, and although she was taking eight drugs (one for each symptom!), she had been getting steadily worse. Just by talking to her Barbour learned that she ran a boarding-house with six boarders to support herself, her alcoholic husband, and a thirty-year-old delinquent, unemployed son. She worked from 5 A.M. to midnight; her only satisfaction derived from her big vegetable garden and the flowers in front of the house. Barbour concludes: "[O]bviously she was exhausted—physically, emotionally, spiritually" (39). Once the process became apparent to doctor and patient, Orvieta was "able to laugh a little about the absurdity of what she expected of herself" (39), and to Barbour's amazement the outcome was a virtual disappearance of her symptoms and a reduction of her drugs to two.

These patients have one thing in common: from the strictly medical point of view they have no identifiable disease. To the dismay of their physicians, their often multiple symptoms and their test results defy diagnosis into a recognizable syndrome. The consequent impasse has been vividly evoked by George Engel, an internist with a psychological bent who practiced in Rochester, New York: "[P]hysicians feel bewildered, inept, frustrated, and angry when sophisticated instrumentation fails to yield answers," while patients for their part feel "used, abused, and dehumanized and become resentful of physicians."[1] Nor is the classification of hypochondriasis apposite, for "the essential feature of hypochondriasis is preoccupation with fears of having, or the idea that one has, a serious disease based on misinterpretation of one or more bodily signs or symptoms."[2] It is not fear of disease that dogs Barbour's patients but diverse relentless pains and disabilities as real to them as they are refractory to treatment by drugs or surgery. So, in the words that Barbour hears from doctors who are themselves "ill at ease with a patient who has no disease," "[H]ow can a patient complain of a sickness when there is 'nothing wrong'?" (37).

The cases Barbour cites suggest the erroneousness of the claim that there is "nothing wrong," in a wider sense despite the absence of demonstrable disease. Barbour's plea for a more broadly based model of caring for patients grows out of his experience that many illnesses are "caused predominantly by personal situations" (1). He argues that "the sick person, not a disease, is the reality" (36). Barbour is careful to emphasize the distinction between disease as a pathological reality, evident in abnormal test findings, and illnesses as expressions of human predicaments that must be explored in their context in order to uncover "the life situation that molded the illness in its present form" (36). Therefore, once actual disease has been ruled out, the focus must be on "patients as persons in family and social systems" (3), for, as Barbour's series of cases reveals, interactions between individuals and the social systems in which they are embedded, may well turn out to underlie their illnesses, especially if tension, hostility, resentment, or even just bewilderment are involved.[3]

Joseph, Jean, Ruth, and Orvieta, together with many others, male and female, whose stories Barbour tells, have psychosomatic disorders. These illnesses are "'idioms of distress' that are employed to express concerns about a broad range of personal and social problems."[4] This basic definition recurs in medical textbooks in varying terms, all of which underscore the role of the physical symptoms as carriers of psychological meaning. For example, Zbigniew Lipowski, a leading researcher in the field, envisages "'psychosomatic' symptoms" as representing "the *preferred* mode of experiencing, expressing, and/or reporting psychological distress."[5] Similarly, the *Synopsis of Psychiatry* designates this kind of symptomatology as "a type of social communication" that may serve "to avoid obligations" such as a disagreeable job, "to express emotions" such as anger, or "to symbolize a feeling or belief" through, for instance, "pain in one's gut."[6] The word "symbolize" here indicates the central metaphoric dimension of the illness as a substitute, culturally sanctioned production of feelings that the patient may regard as socially prohibited. This displacement of emotion into the body is forefronted in the textbook *Abnormal Psychology*, which explains "psychosomatic" as a manifestation where "the body expresses psychological conflict and stress in unusual, and sometimes bizarre, fashion."[7] The most graphic formulation comes from Susan Sontag, who designates illness as "what speaks through the body, a language for dramatizing the mental as a form of self-expression."[8]

Such dramatization of the mental through the body is known in psychiatry as conversion. It is, in effect, a form of translation, as states of mind are projected into the body, which is made to act as a scapegoat. When emotions are "converted" into symptoms, they are simultaneously masked *and* manifested in a nonverbal style of communication. The recuperation of the covert psychological meaning, the retrieval into verbal utterance (and thus into consciousness) is the essence of Barbour's work with his patients. This naming of the feelings or situations animating the conversion makes it amenable to more rational analysis and thereby extricates it from the body, which is relieved of the task of indirect communication imposed on it in the conversion process.

This principle of a transfer from mind to body underlies the diagnostic criteria for conversion disorder laid down in *DSM-IV*:

A. One or more symptoms or deficits affecting voluntary motor or sensory function which suggest a neurological or other general medical condition.

B. Psychological factors are judged to be associated with the symptom or deficit because the initiation or exacerbation of the symptom or deficit is preceded by conflicts or other stressors.

C. The symptom or deficit is not intentionally produced or feigned (as in Factitious Disorder or Malingering).

D. The symptom or deficit cannot, after appropriate investigation, be fully explained by a general medical condition, or by the direct effects of a substance, or as a culturally sanctioned behavior or experience.

E. The symptom or deficit causes clinically significant distress or impairment in social, occupational, or other important areas of functioning or warrants medical evaluation. (457)

Since conversion disorders can simulate medical conditions of any kind, *DSM-IV* requires specification of the type of symptom or deficit. However, as the extensive testing of Barbour's patients discloses, the symptomatology does not correspond to known syndromes, nor do the laboratory findings indicate abnormalities. "In fact," *DSM-IV* points out, "it is the absence of expected findings that suggests and supports the diagnosis of Conversion Disorder" (455). The implausibility of the symptoms and especially of the symptom combinations in discrete parts of the body may also alert the physician to the possibility of such a disorder. Under these circumstances, psychological factors have to be probed. It is their role as stressors in initiating and exacerbating the physical symptoms that is crucial for the appearance of psychosomatic disorders as language in the body.

In practice the distinction between disease and illness may not be nearly as categoric as Barbour's clear-cut examples imply. Disease is described as "organic" because it stems from changes in the *structure* of bodily tissues that can be visualized through X rays, MRIs, or CAT scans or that become manifest as abnormalities in bodily fluids. The term complementary to "organic" is "functional," which denotes the absence of such pathological changes and consequently attributes the complaint to a disturbance in *function*. These two words have tended to be used as a means of discriminating between somatic and psychosomatic symptoms. As recently as 1997 Steven L. Dubovsky stated in *Mind-Body Deceptions*: "Symptoms that cannot be traced to identifiable somatic problems are called functional complaints because they are a function of a psychological process and not a product of a structural change in the tissues of the body" (91). Such a distinction reaches back to an earlier tradition. Franz Alexander, a Freudian who wrote on psychosomatic disorders from the 1930s to the 1950s, for a while favored the dissociation of "organic" and "functional." The differentiation is indeed legitimate: a headache may be due to annoyance or to a brain tumor; in the latter case, it is likely to be persistent, progresively severe, and detectable by modern technology; on the other hand, if it is a precipitate of annoyance, it will probably dissipate spontaneously and fairly quickly. But Alexander himself in his major book, *Psychosomatic Medicine* (1950), acknowledged that "nature does not know such strict distinctions as 'functional' versus 'organic'" (43).

So the former division into organic and nonorganic disturbances "is gradually disappearing."[9] That concession was made in 1988 by Benjamin Wolman, author of *Psychosomatic Disorders*. Eleven years later the same view was voiced with far greater bluntness, when John C. Marshall, a neuropsychologist at the Radcliffe Infirmary, Oxford, asserted point-blank that "no one believes in the mind-body dualism any more, and hence the old distinction between functional and organic conditions can no longer be drawn."[10] Even *DSM-IV*, which, as a diagnostic manual aims to achieve utmost delineations, issues the warning that "[i]t is important to note, however, that conversion symptoms can occur in individuals with neurological conditions" (455). The estimate given is that "as many as one third of individuals with conversion symptoms have a current or prior neurological condition" (453). A still higher figure, one half, is cited in *Abnormal Psychology* (239–40) for patients treated for a psychosomatic disorder who receive a subsequent medical diagnosis. Similarly, the *Synopsis of Psychiatry* found systemic disease of the brain prior or concomitantly in 18 to 64 percent of hospitalized patients with conversion disorders, and nonpsychiatric disorders are eventually diagnosed in 25 to 50 percent of them (623). These numbers suggest, first, that even the most up-to-date diagnostic methods are far from infallible, and second, that there is a tendency to assume that symptoms in certain segments of the population are more likely to be psychosomatic. It is no coincidence that Barbour's patients comprise conspicuously more women than men.[11]

Recognition of this overlap between organic and functional, between disease and illness complicates the diagnosis of psychosomatic disorders. "Functional or 'psychosomatic' symptoms may occur in the presence or absence of demonstrable organic disease," Lipowski notes.[12] Barbour plays down this overlap for the sake of the incisiveness of his argument, although he is well aware of the interplay not only between mind and body but also between disease and illness: "[T]he disease itself can be accentuated by ongoing emotional disturbance in some patients" (50). Certain diseases, notably asthma, hypertension, and heart conditions are particularly liable to be affected by emotional disturbances.

As a corollary to the waning of the old opposition between organic and functional, the role of psychological factors in the processes of drift from dysfunction to structural disease has attracted increasing attention. Alexander already observed that "local anatomical changes themselves may result from more general disturbances which develop in consequence of faulty function, excessive stress, or even emotional factors."[13] Functional disorders of long duration may gradually lead to serious organic disorders associated with morphological changes. The mechanisms conducive to such changes have been spelled out in varied but broadly consensual terms in recent medical writing; for example, "[W]hen an intense stress provoking stimulus ('stressor') acts on an organism, the organism responds by a series of biochemical and physiological changes in the glands of inner secretion, called the 'alarm reaction.' The alarm reaction is followed by increased hormonal secretion of the pituitary gland, which activates the cortex of the adrenal gland."[14] Or, as another writer explains, a vulnerable organ subjected to ongoing stress may be permanently changed: "Once the heart adjusts to beating at an excessive rate, or the blood vessels remain in spasm long enough, the affected system may reset itself to a pathological level of functioning that is independent of the emotional state that originally mobilized it."[15] So disturbed function can actually lead to disturbed structure. The emotional conflicts that cause continued fluctuations in blood pressure can, in the long run, result in chronically elevated blood pressure and irreversible forms of kidney damage. Or a sustained paralysis of a limb, found to be without pathological foundation and therefore deemed psychosomatic, will through sheer inactivity trigger degenerative changes in muscles and joints.

One consequence of this abandonment of the radical separation of organic and functional is the tendency to claim the involvement of psychological factors in all sickness. Advocates of this position declare "that social and psychological factors play some role in the predisposition to, initiation of, response to, and maintenance of every disease."[16] Such beliefs are based partly on research in immunology, specifically into the forces

that strengthen or lower an individual's immune system. That those who
have sustained a loss or who are suffering from depression are more liable
to infections and other kinds of ill-health has long been known. Before
advances in immunology, attempts were made to establish direct connections between psychological and physical processes and to link certain diseases to particular emotions. Tuberculosis was thought to stem from an
excess of passion and cancer conversely from the repression of passion.
Herself a cancer survivor, Sontag protests vehemently against these simpli-
fications of the mind-body relationship: "[T]he hypothesis that distress can
affect immunological response (and, in some circumstances, lower immu-
nity to disease) is hardly the same as—or constitutes evidence for—the view
that emotions cause diseases, much less that specific emotions can produce
specific diseases."[17] Sontag's lay views are supported by Lipowski's considered medical assessment: "It is meaningless to say that emotions cause disease; they cause nothing. It is equally incorrect to propose that any other
psychological variable causes disease; it can only influence susceptibility to
disease through the mediation of neuroendocrine processes controlled by
the brain."[18] The key word here is "susceptibility," which fashions a judicious bridge between "emotions" and "neuroendocrine processes."

The confluence of the functional and the organic is of enormous
importance for the approach to psychosomatic disorders, although it
greatly magnifies the difficulties of both medical diagnosis and cognitive
understanding. For the slippage places psychosomatic disorders in the borderlands between pronounced physical pathologies and psychological
problems. So their intrinsic elusiveness is vastly heightened. To compound
the problem further, psychosomatic medicine lacks a site anchored in any
one area of the body in the way that cardiology, gastroenterology, nephrol-
ogy, or dermatology do. Since psychosomatic disorders can surface in any
part of the body, they hover homelessly in shadowlands; not localized, they
are potentially everywhere, yet also nowhere. Shifting and at times poly-
symptomatic, they exhibit a peculiar vagrancy that is at once their hallmark
and a primary source of the puzzlement they occasion.

Because of this instability, malattributions and misdiagnoses in regard
to psychosomatic disorders are not surprising. Even with the latest tech-
nologies misconstructions are not unusual. To revert to Barbour's patients,
Orvieta, for instance, had collected working diagnoses of irritable-bowel
syndrome, tension headaches, lumbosacral strain syndrome, bursitis, neuralgia, and asthma. With disarming honesty Barbour adds, "I found myself
in general agreement with the prevailing diagnoses,"[19] before heeding her
life situation and realizing that the overarching clue to her complaints lay
in her exhaustion. Before the technological advances of the past hundred
and fifty years or so, differential diagnosis was infinitely more difficult, not
to say virtually impossible until the autopsy. For instance, toward the end of

the nineteenth century, Pierre Janet, the eminent French psychologist, observed a fourteen-year-old girl admitted to hospital with apparently neurotic symptoms; when she died soon afterward, the postmortem revealed a hydatic cyst on the brain.[20] The neurotic origin of general paralysis was disproven by the discovery in 1913 by H. Noguchin and J. W. Moore of the microorganism *treponema pallidum,* which pointed to the syphilitic causation of some paralyses.[21] Pseudoseizures are distinguishable from genuine seizures by means of at least two criteria: the pupillary and gag reflexes are retained in pseudoseizures, and no postseizure increase in prolactin concentrations is found in blood tests. The establishment of the biological bases of epilepsy, in fact, led to its transfer from psychiatry to neurology.

The history of medicine confirms Sontag's assertion that "theories that diseases are caused by mental states and can be cured by will power are always an index of how little is understood about the physical terrain of the disease."[22] A case in point is chronic fatigue syndrome: current opinion oscillates between the hypothesis of a viral etiology, on the grounds that some antibodies are elevated in some patients' blood, or its categorization as a psychosomatic disorder.[23] While medical advances have mostly fostered more precise diagnoses and the transfer of syndromes from the vague, capacious segment of emotionally caused disturbances, the crossover may also take place in the opposite direction. Hiram Houston Merritt's *Textbook of Neurology* does not use the term "psychosomatic," but it does suggest psychotherapy as a treatment for some cases of migraine (628–29), thereby tacitly conceding the possibility of psychological origins.

The potential for vastly differing interpretations of the same symptomatology is at the heart of Flannery O'Connor's amusing and ironic story "The Enduring Chill." Asbury, an aspiring playwright, comes back to his southern home from New York with attacks of fever. His mother, who meets him at the train, gives a little involuntary cry as she glimpses his shockingly sick appearance and his bloodshot eyes. Perversely, he is "pleased that she should see death in his face at once" (110). For "he had felt the end coming on for nearly four months. Alone in his freezing flat, huddled under his two blankets and his overcoat, with three thicknesses of the New York *Times* between, he had had a chill one night, followed by a violent sweat that left the sheets soaking and removed all doubt from his mind about his true condition" (110). After his return, his rapid decline continues. So convinced is he of his imminent death that he has the priest come. He looks out toward the pasture, where his grave will be, and visualizes his funeral. His mother, in what seems like denial, thinks he is having "a nervous breakdown" (113), while his sister scoffingly blames his illness on his failure at writing. Asbury drafts a self-explanatory letter to his mother that fills two notebooks. Much of "The Enduring Chill" is devoted to exposition of the tense family dynamics between mother, son, and daughter, thereby hinting at a psychological source for Asbury's illness. He refuses to let the local family doctor, Block, come to see him: "'What's wrong with me,' he repeated, 'is way beyond Block'" (113). Finally, in alarm, his strong-willed mother insists on bringing in the country doctor, who cheerfully counters Asbury's protest, "'What's wrong with me is way beyond you'" with "'Most things are beyond me.—I ain't found anything yet that I thoroughly understand'"(121). Thanks to a blood sample Dr. Block diagnoses undulating fever. Disobeying his mother, Asbury had drunk unpasteurized milk, an act of defiance whose rashness is underscored by the black farm hands' refusal to do likewise. The artist's psychosomatic illness unto death is unmasked as a foolish, risk-taking behavior that had caused a physical disease.

So "What Does the Word 'Psychosomatic' Really Mean?" Lipowski asks in an article written in 1984.[24] Though a sound starting point for exploration of the field, the article does not provide any categoric answers. Its title, consisting of a query, suggests a quest rather than conclusions, a point confirmed by its subtitle, "A Historical and Semantic Inquiry."

Lipowski's inquiry was prompted by the questions that students, colleagues, and lay people frequently asked him not only about the meaning of the term but also about the scope of the field. The mere necessity for such questions in itself already testifies to the perplexity intrinsic to the concept. Lacking clearly delineated limits, "psychosomatic" runs the risk of amorphousness, like nineteenth-century "neurasthenia." "Psychosomatic" itself was first used in 1818 by a professor of psychiatry in Leipzig, Johann Christian August Heinroth, who applied it to insomnia.

Nor do dictionary definitions help with "psychosomatic"; on the contrary they create more problems than they solve because they raise the extremely tricky issue of the mind-body relationship. *Webster's* dictionary gives "(a) of or pertaining to those bodily symptoms which arise from or are traceable to mental conditions; (b) pertaining to both body and mind as a single entity." The word did not make its way into the *Oxford English Dictionary* until a 1982 supplement, where it appeared as an adjective: "involving or depending on both the mind and the body as mutually dependent entities." *Medical Meanings,* refers to the derivation from "psycho-" plus Greek *soma,* "the body," to arrive at the description: "whatever has an integral mind-body relationship." The *Synopsis of Psychiatry* gracefully sidesteps too ready a definition by envisaging "psychosomatic" as a diagnosis that "reflects the clinician's assessment that psychological factors are a large contributor to the symptoms' onset, severity, and duration" (617). *DSM-IV* opts for an exclusionary method by endorsing the criterion that "psychosomatic" denotes those complaints for which an adequate medical explanation cannot be found.

Medical textbooks, on the other hand, eschew the problem of the mind-body relationship. Lipowski dismisses as "rather facile" the discussions that "have raged about its alleged metaphysical connotations, that is, whether it [psychosomatic medicine] affirmed the unity or duality of mind and body."[25] Such meditations, he says, are avoided in the medical arena as belonging to theology and philosophy. In the last resort, the interface between mind and body remains uncharted territory despite momentous advances in medicine. For instance, with many of the newest psychotropic drugs experimentation proves that they work for some patients, but their precise mechanisms are not known. Evidence shows that while the mind-body relationship is a potent force, it is not as yet fully amenable to rational understanding. The authors of *Abnormal Psychology*, for example, cite the connection between an important exam and an upset stomach or a headache. Observation and experience bear out the incidence of such a correlation; indeed it is so common as to be rarely scrutinized. Yet, the authors admit, it is "not easily explained" (248); they conclude that "the translation from 'mind' to 'body' occurs in a way that defies medical logic" (238). Thus the proposition that the psyche may speak through the body has attained widespread acceptance, although the pathways of this process remain in many respects mysterious.

The difficulty of discovering "what the word 'psychosomatic' really means" therefore hinges on the much deeper underlying problem of the mind-body relationship. Medical writers have repeatedly, even in the past twenty years, conceded the impasse in varying terminology. "The final answer is still a controversial issue," Wolman acknowledges, and the term "psychosomatic" itself "quite ambiguous."[26] In his 1982 survey of "Contemporary Research and the Mind-Body Problem" Weiner concedes that psychosomatic medicine is often critized for not being able to offer an answer to the question how "social experience and/or psychological conflicts and induced emotions could be possibly translated (transduced) into bodily physiology leading to illness" (223). To some extent the recognition of the confluence of functional and organic has mapped some of the intermediary steps in such a process of conversion, but without addressing the ultimate enigma of the mind-body interaction.

Of all those who have sought to define "psychosomatic" Lipowski is both the most outspoken and the most authoritative. He does not shun indeterminacy or even a rather negative response to his own query, "What Does the Word 'Psychosomatic' Really Mean?" Indeed, "really" comes across as almost ironic in light of Lipowski's statement: "The meaning of the term 'psychosomatic medicine' remains unclear and no generally agreed upon definition of it exists."[27] Equally direct is his assertion that "the field of psychosomatic medicine abounds in semantic and conceptual confusion. There is no general agreement regarding the meaning of basic terms, not enough distinction between what are data of observation and theoretical concepts and explanatory hypotheses, and little consensus about the scope of the discipline and its position within the larger fields of medicine, psychiatry, and human biology" (27). Lipowski judges the word to mean "no more than we agree that it should mean, and we delimit its boundaries by defining it" (4). He also warns that "sharp delineation of the field [is] difficult if not actually undesirable" (133). In arguing against sharp delineation—and so by implication in favor of a certain openness— Lipowski goes against the mainstream of somatic medicine, which aspires to exact diagnoses, and moves psychosomatic medicine toward a more pronouncedly humanistic mode. That, of course, is exactly what Barbour learned to do with his patients.

Nevertheless, Lipowski does not stop at mere demonstration of the misguidedness of pursuing a definitive meaning of "psychosomatic." He argues that psychosomatic medicine has to insist on "the inseparability of mind and body as well as their mutual dependence" (120). So it must affirm an "antidualistic stance" (120), perceiving mind and body as one or as only separate aspects of a person or an organism as a whole. The fundamental outlook of psychosomatics is therefore essentially "*holistic*" (120) in contradistinction to the fragmentation of late twentieth- and early twenty-first-century somatic medicine, with its system of specialties and subspecialties. The definition that Lipowski proposes toward the end of his article underscores the holism that he sees as the core connotation: "*Psychosomatic* is a term referring or related to the inseparability and interdependence of psychosocial and biologic (physiologic, somatic) aspects of humankind" (133). He goes on:

> *Psychosomatic medicine* (psychosomatics) refers to a discipline concerned with (1) the study of the correlation of psychologic and social phenomena with physiologic functions . . . , and of the interplay of biologic and psychosocial factors in the development, course, and outcome of diseases; and (2) advocacy of a holistic (or biopsychosocial) approach to patient care and application of methods derived from behavioral sciences to the prevention and treatment of human morbidity. (133)

In defining psychosomatics Lipowski uses a term that has been assuming increasing prominence and that comes as close to the "meaning" of psychosomatic as is feasible: "biopsychosocial." He introduces the term in quotes at the opening of his article, where he expresses the hope that it may replace "psychosomatic" because it is free of "the ambiguity and controversy" (119) that continue to surround "psychosomatic."[28]

"Biopsychosocial" is a term first launched by George Engel in a series of articles published in the late 1970s and early 1980s. Engel takes care to spell out the angle from which he comes to psychosomatics: "[M]y training and personal identity is that of an internist with special interest in its psychosomatic and psychosocial aspects. I have had no formal psychiatric training and have never had a psychiatric practice. I have tried to achieve the level of competence in psychiatry than any competent physician should have."[29] It is his experience in internal medicine that convinces him (like Barbour, later) of the absolute necessity of heeding dimensions beyond just the biological in the treatment of disease.

Engel's key example, which he elaborates in detail in an article in the *American Journal of Psychiatry* in 1980, "The Clinical Application of the Biopsychosocial Model," and to which he refers in succeeding publications, is that of Mr. Glover, a fifty-five-year old married real estate agent with two adult sons, who is brought to the hospital with symptoms similar to those he had experienced six months earlier when he had had a heart attack. He responds well at first to the prompt institution of coronary care, but thirty minutes later, in the midst of the continuing workup, he abruptly loses consciousness and goes into ventricular fibrillation. After successful defibrillation, Mr. Glover makes an uneventful recovery.

Engel analyzes what happened in this case from two parallel but distinct perspectives: the biomedical and the biopsychosocial. The normative biomedical model, which is followed in the hospital, is by far the simpler: "For the reductionist physician a diagnosis of 'acute myocardial infarction' suffices to characterize Mr. Glover's problem and to define the doctor's job. Indeed, once so categorized Mr. Glover is likely to be referred to by the staff as 'an MI'" (538). Engel criticizes this routine method as reductionist because it is predicated on the premise that the cause of Mr. Glover's complaints and the requirements for his care can be localized to the injury to the tissues, cells, and molecules of one particular organ. In this scenario the patient's feelings and reactions are given virtually no attention. The aim of the dominant biomedical model—to diagnose and treat the disease as quickly as possible—encourages neglect of psychosocial dimensions, which may turn out to be decisive. There is no better illustration of this tendency than Barbour's patients, with their multiple diagnoses, drugs, and surgeries as a direct consequence of neglect of elements in their lives beyond the strictly medical.

By contrast, the biopsychosocial model envisages Mr. Glover not only as a person with a damaged heart but also as an individual within a family and a community. Engel emphasizes that "*[i]n the continuity of natural systems every unit is at the very same time both a whole and a part*" (537). So the patient may be importantly influenced by processes at the psychological and inter-personal levels of organization. Mr. Glover, for example, initially denies the seriousness of his symptoms, specifically, the possibility of another heart attack; although aware of the similarity of his symptoms to those of his ear-lier heart attack, he prefers to see them as fatigue, or muscle strain, or indi-gestion, or emotional tension. He stays at work, alternating between sitting quietly at his desk and pacing the office; he avoids other employees, and takes Alka-Seltzer. Engel interprets Mr. Glover's behavior as an expression of complex feelings: fear of losing his job and control over his own destiny as well as an assertion of his personal values of responsibility and inde-pendence. Only the intervention of his employer enables him to accept the need for hospitalization and patient status. The psychological stabilization attendant on this decision has stabilizing effects on other systems too, so that by the time Mr. Glover reaches the hospital, he no longer has chest pains and feels relatively calm and confident.

What then precipitates his dangerous relapse when he is already under medical care? Engel attributes it to a massive rise in Mr. Glover's anxiety, coincident with his loss of confidence in the competence of the medical staff, which is prompted by the house officer's difficulty in drawing arterial blood. Such difficulty is not uncommon, as arteries are elastic and tend to jump away at the touch of a needle. For the uninformed patient the ten-minute unproductive efforts to carry out this procedure are painful, dis-agreeable, distressing, even frightening. When the house officer leaves to fetch help, Mr. Glover feels let down by the medical personnel whom he had trusted as powerful to help him. Now instead, he feels victimized by inexperienced physicians, and angry at having allowed himself to become entrapped in this predicament. Blaming himself, he has a growing sense of helplessness. Concomitantly he gets hot and flushed, and the chest pain returns. These are the circumstances under which the life-threatening ven-tricular fibrillation sets in.

Engel contends, convincingly, that the difficulty over the arterial punc-ture should have been recognized early as a risk for the patient, not just a technical problem for a junior doctor. Mr. Glover's failure to complain should also have been recognized as characteristic of his psychological style of denial rather than as an untroubled acquiescence. In short, the episode of the ventricular fibrillation could have been avoided if an inclusive approach had been taken that took into account Mr. Glover's feelings and reactions, his conflicts about hospitalization and his anxieties about the implications for his work and family of his repeated heart attacks.

Engel seeks to win acceptance of the biopsychosocial model by presenting it as a scientific one. He charts the reciprocal interactions of the psychological and the physiological during the fruitless attempts at arterial puncture and the subsequent cardiac arrest (figs. 5 and 6, 540). He readily grants that the example of Mr. Glover is an "oversimplification" (543), although his arguments for the mutual interdependence of the patient's feelings and his heart condition are persuasive. More problematical is Engel's advocacy of the clinical application of the biopsychosocial model in an emergency situation such as an acute heart attack. The imperative for speed in delivering immediate care is likely to result in the setting aside of any investigation of the patient's psychological style and social environment in favor of more urgent needs. The biopsychosocial model becomes wholly appropriate, however, in the context of Barbour's Diagnostic Clinic, to which the cases most resistant to diagnosis are referred and where rapidity is no longer a primary concern.

Whatever the obstacles to the application of the biopsychosocial model in the emergency room, it is without doubt ideally suited to the analysis of illness in literary characters. For while the literary work is inevitably weak on those kinds of quantitative information on which modern medicine relies so heavily, it compensates for this shortfall by qualitative strength in the density of the characters' psychological traits and their social environment. Novels, short stories, and plays normally show the context of the action, the circumstances that lead to the choice of one course over another, and the motivation for behaviors. Their spatial and temporal expansiveness creates a forum for the portrayal of interpersonal relationships as they develop over a period of days, months, or often years. Family conflicts, stresses arising from work, the impact on individuals of their physical and human surroundings, sources of guilt, the see-saw of losses and gains, evasions, deprivations, frustrations, and hurts: all these form the subject matter of literature, and all are highly conducive to the elaboration of the dynamics of psychosomatic disorders.

The aptitude of literature for the in-depth representation of illness is best illustrated by imagining Mr. Glover as a figure not in a medical article but in a novel. Engel himself engages in some speculation as part of his plea for greater heed to the patient's social environment. He maintains, for instance, that the "continuity of systems makes attention to Mrs. Glover's well-being a necessary element in Mr. Glover's care" (543) for if Mrs. Glover were to suffer a breakdown or illness, or even death, Mr. Glover's prospects would be affected too.

The introduction of Mrs. Glover opens up large vistas for the literary imagination onto a medley of factors that could have been instrumental in precipitating Mr. Glover's two heart attacks. In a novel or play the nature of the marriage could have been exposed: Was it a Strindbergian battle of the sexes? Was Mrs. Glover a nagging wife, goading her husband to better their lives by making more money? Were there sexual problems such as impotence on the part of the aging man? Had a dirty secret recently been brought to light? Had some life-sustaining illusion long cherished by the Glovers been shattered? Does Mr. Glover like his work in the real estate office? Does he get on well with his colleagues, or does competition for listings and sales foster rivalries and animosities? Does Mr. Glover have a tendency to, or even a history of depression? Does he harbor grudges or is he forgiving? Does Mrs. Glover work? Does she enjoy it for the companionship, or does she resent it as a reminder of her husband's inadequacy as the family's breadwinner? And what about the two adult sons? Do they give their parents satisfaction or grief? Are they committed to respectable work, or in jail? What are their marriages like? Do the Glovers like their daughters-in-law? Are there grandchildren? Are they a source of pleasure or of worry to their grandparents? Does Mr. or Mrs. Glover have an aged parent who imposes the strain of constant vigilance as well as a financial drain?

These various facets of Mr. Glover's social context and psychological profile could be depicted in a literary work to fill out his entire history leading up to the heart attacks. His life would be interpreted as a series of responses at crucial junctures, largely conditioned by his upbringing, his previous experiences, and his disposition. The biological event of the "MI" would be seen as the outcome of a lengthy, complicated psychosocial development. For literature presents characters in the way in which Joseph Sapira, in his 1992 presidential address to the American Psychosomatic Society, argues that patients should be viewed: "Patients not only exist as collections of organs, cells, molecules, ions, and so forth but also as individuals and members of romantic dyads, families, geographic units, language clans, religious units, sexes, ethnic groups, nations, and so forth. Furthermore, they bring to any illness situation their past individual experiences as total organisms whose individual histories cannot be grasped by an exclusively reductionist approach."[30] The questions that Sapira urges doctors to ask patients about their lives as individuals are precisely those that Barbour put to his patients—and that literary works ask and answer. The humanistic vision of literature has the capacity to offer a rich etiology of the psychosomatic illness along biopsychosocial lines by exploring how the patient comes to be driven to speak through the body.

CHAPTER TWO

Swings of the Historical Pendulum

Patient: "The heart is on the left and the liver on the right."
Doctor: "Yes, that was so in the old days. But we have changed all that."
—Molière, *Le medecin malgré lui*

"Until the mid-nineteenth century, . . . , all medicine was necessarily and ubiquitously 'psychosomatic,'" the eminent medical historian Charles Rosenberg asserts in his incisive article "Mind and Body in Nineteenth-Century Medicine" (77). "Every clinician," he goes on, "had to be something of a psychiatrist and family therapist" (78). So the necessity for a comprehensive view that Barbour learns with his perplexing patients and that Engel posits in his biopsychosocial model was intrinsic to medicine up to the mid-nineteenth century. The holistic mode was so much a matter of course that "there was no need for a special term to describe the unquestioned common sense of perceived experience."[1] Nor was there much need for the word "psychosomatic" because the style of medicine it denotes was the norm.

Rosenberg's statements raise two major questions that will be addressed in this chapter: Why was medicine "necessarily" psychosomatic until the mid-nineteenth century? And what happened at that period to eclipse the system of beliefs and practices that had up to that point supported this approach? A brief look at the history of medicine reveals the swings of the pendulum from holistic to somatic, and then at least some way back again. The movements of this pendulum were not regular; for centuries it was almost stationary, then it moved conspicuously from one pole to the other and then gradually returned part of the way, at least among some practitioners.

Medicine was "necessarily" psychosomatic from classical antiquity into the nineteenth century because its cornerstone from the time of Galen, a Greek physician born in A.D. 130, was the theory of the four "humors." The universe was recognized as consisting of four elements: earth, air, water, and fire. These were thought to correspond in the human body to cold, dry, moist, and hot humors. Good health was believed to result from the proper balance of the humors; when one or another got the upper hand, the appropriate corrective was to resort to its opposite, applying heat to cold areas and vice versa, and treating dryness and moisture as parallel counteragents. Very important, this doctrine extended too to the individual's psychological profile, for each person was held to be endowed with a preponderance of one humor or another, resulting in a sanguine, phlegmatic, choleric, or melancholic temperament respectively.

The first step toward remediating a humoral imbalance was to establish the patient's distinctive humor. Then the chosen therapy was tailored to fit the particular patient in light of his or her dominant humor, age, and situation, that is, the time of year, the climate, the location, and so on. Two patients with identical symptoms might be given quite divergent treatments because of the perceived differences in their circumstances. Thus the outcome of humoral medicine was patient-specific treatment whose primary aim was to restore the individual's natural homeostasis.

This form of therapeutics rested on a close and extensive familiarity with the whole person on the physician's part in order to achieve an encompassing cure. Attention had to be paid to the emotions as an essential facet of the patient's temperament likely to determine the outcome. In other words, psyche and soma were not regarded as distinct entities. Clinical observation confirmed the supposition of the reciprocal interaction between mind and body: "The fact that bodily diseases and symptoms are profoundly influenced by mental processes, often partially caused by them, was well known to all great clinicians from Galen to Charcot."[2] Accordingly, medicine was holistic and empirical, drawing on experience to buttress humoral theory. The danger to the entire organism of uncontrolled feelings was a basic tenet of humoral medicine: "[E]motions out of balance meant physiological function out of balance."[3] So "psychogenesis, or 'passion-produced disease,' as Galen called it, was discussed abundantly until the nineteenth century."[4]

This view marks the full swing of the pendulum toward the total integration of mind and body. By and large it maintained its ascendancy until the nineteenth century, making medicine "ubiquitously 'psychosomatic,'" as Rosenberg puts it, and "necessarily" so, partly for lack of detailed knowledge of the workings of mind or body that would challenge the speculative theories of humoral medicine. This is not to minimize the fundamental progress made between the sixteenth to eighteenth centuries by such researchers as Andreas Vesalius (1514–64), who mapped human anatomy; William Harvey (1578–1616), who expounded the circulation of blood; and Giovanni Morgagni (1682–1771), who made the first attempt to relate clinical symptoms to findings at autopsies. But these early medical advances did not prejudice the acceptance of a connection between mind and body, based on accumulated empirical evidence.

The gravest threat to the holistic approach came from an entirely different quarter, from the philosophy of René Descartes (1596–1650), a mathematician who sought in his *Discours de la méthode* (1637; Discourse on Method) to extend the logical method to all branches of knowledge. His programmatic doubt of everything other than the reasoning power of his own mind led him to formulate the proposition "Cogito, ergo sum" (I think, therefore I am) as the only trustworthy foundation for his philosophy. Through its distinction between being and thinking, this proposition implies a de facto split between mind and body.

However, medical opinion continued to affirm the unity of psyche and soma well into the nineteenth century; diagnostics and therapeutics alike were "integrated, with psyche and soma as part of the same system of pathology."[5] Expressions of belief in such integration crop up frequently between the seventeenth and mid-nineteenth century. Thomas Sydenham (1624–89), the preeminent British physician of his time, declared that psychological factors were involved in pathogenesis. In the latter half of the eighteenth century a series of monographs appeared that sought to offer a systematic presentation of contemporary views of the influence of the mind upon the body. William Corp's *Essay on the Changes Produced in the Body by Operations of the Mind* (1791) and William Falconer's *Dissertation on the Influence of the Passions upon Disorders of the Body* (1796) discuss both the deleterious and the beneficial effects of the mental faculties. Thoughts and emotions such as hope, joy, anger, fear, grief, and anxiety were recognized as having a direct impact on physical conditions.

Outstanding among these treatises are the two essays published under the title *De regime mentis* (1747 and 1763) by Jerome Gaub (1705–80), a professor of medicine at Leiden whose work was widely known in the eighteenth century. In considering the question of the relation of body to mind in human ailments, Gaub presented clearly, forcefully, and often elegantly a summary of current opinion. His opening section, "The Harmony of Mind and Body" (34), places him squarely in the tradition of humoral medicine. The crucial role of the interplay of mind and body in health and sickness forms the recurrent motif in such essays as "Mind-Body Interaction in the Normal State" (48–53), "Mind-Body Interaction in States of Disturbance" (53–59), and "Corporeal Effects of Expressed and Suppressed

Emotions Compared" (180–83). Gaub argues that if emotions "irrupt on the surface in such number and profusion, think how much more violently the interior parts where they arise must be disturbed" (132). Gaub's advocacy of the mind-body dynamic is impressive. He ends by stating that he has "made it quite plain that the causes and occasions of a great many affections of the body arise in the mind, as it were from a fountainhead" (195). Almost two hundred and fifty years later Barbour in his advanced Diagnostic Clinic at Stanford Medical Center would reach much the same conclusion.

The interdependence of mind and body was also acclaimed by powerful voices in the late eighteenth and early nineteenth centuries. Pierre Cabanis (1750–1808), a highly influential French physician, warned in 1797: "Woe to the medical man who has not learned to read the human heart as well as to recognize the febrile state."[6] A parallel view was expressed by Benjamin Rush (1745–1813), the most prominent American physician of his day: "Man is said to be a compound of soul and body. However proper this language may be in religion, it is not so in medicine. He is, in the eye of a physician, a single and indivisible being, for so intimately united are his soul and body, that one cannot be moved, without the other."[7]

As late as the mid-nineteenth century, medical writing still strongly suggests an awareness of a class of disorders that would later come to be identified as psychosomatic. In the section "Obligations of Patients to Their Physicians" in the 1847 Code of Ethics adopted by the American Medical Association, patients are admonished "faithfully and unreservedly" to "communicate to their physician the supposed cause of their disease. This is the more important, as many diseases of a mental origin simulate those depending on external causes, and yet are only to be cured by ministering to the mind diseased."[8] These instructions come remarkably close to an acknowledgment of the principle underlying psychosomatic conversion. In a similar vein, the French physician Michel Lévy writes in 1844 of patients who complain of "des sensations les plus pénibles et les plus étranges" (most painful and peculiar sensations), "de souffrances aussi mobiles par leur siège que difficiles à caractériser" (symptoms as mobile in their location as difficult to characterize). These patients' puzzling symptomatology, he notes, causes them panic and despair as they complain at times about their head, at others about their stomach.[9] Although Lévy does not discuss the psychological processes involved, he aptly outlines a profile of psychosomatic disorders on the basis of his observations.

By the mid-nineteenth century, cases that seem to be psychosomatic in origin appear in literary works. Most conspicuous is the large number of mysterious "brain fevers" that suddenly befall characters. The best known of the literary figures prey to this affliction around the middle of the century are Catherine Linton in Emily Brontë's *Wuthering Heights* (1847),[10] Emma in Flaubert's *Madame Bovary* (1857), Pip in Dickens's *Great Expectations* (1860), and Roghozin in Dostoevsky's *The Idiot* (1868).[11] Although these dangerous, potentially fatal attacks are presented in a predominantly physical guise as consisting of high fever, prostration, and loss of consciousness, they generally follow a violent nervous shock, thereby at least suggesting a psychological component.[12]

Apart from these dramatic illnesses, subtler instances of the interaction of mind and body surface around mid-century too. Balzac's *Le Cousin Pons* (1847), hailed by Alexander as "one of the first psychosomatic novels ever written,"[13] traces the decline and death of Pons, a musician whose health is seriously undermined by his discovery late in life of the vicious greed and betrayal of the very people who had posed as his friends. Echoing and underscoring the fate of Pons is that of his one true friend, who succumbs to a stroke within a few days of realizing how he has likewise been outwitted and cheated of his inheritance. The repetition of the same fatal outcome after a severe emotional shock testifies to the conjunction of mind and body.

Even more extensive coverage of psychosomatic disorders occurs in Charlotte Brontë's *Shirley* (1849), which portrays four cases of illness, all of which in some way fuse soma and psyche. The hero, Robert Moore, a factory owner, goes through a period of depression during his lengthy recovery from a gunshot wound inflicted by disaffected workmen at the time of the industrial revolution: "I am hopelessly weak, and the state of my mind is inexpressible—dark, barren, impotent."[14] The governess-companion, Mrs. Pryor, in recounting her life story, also recalls how at one point she "sickened" for "want of affection" (298). Shirley herself goes into a kind of decline after being bitten by a dog; she looks pale and sad, grows thin and hollow-eyed out of fear of death from rabies. She withdraws from her friends and makes her will, all the while maintaining silence about her anxieties. When Robert notices her disquiet (which proves unfounded), he urges her to speak out: "Nervous alarms should always be communicated that they may be dissipated" (399). The most serious illness in the novel is that of Shirley's friend, Caroline, who "wasted like any snow-wreath in thaw; faded like any flower in drought" (331). Exhausted by fevers, she believes herself to be physically sick, yet the cause of her "inward wound" proves to be her secret love for Robert and her belief that he is about to marry Shirley. All the main characters in *Shirley* sicken physically, albeit for varying reasons, yet in every instance those reasons are closely related to psychological factors.

The examples of *Le Cousin Pons* and *Shirley*, together with the explicit statements in the medical writings up to the early nineteenth century, corroborate Rosenberg's contention that medicine was "ubiquitously psychosomatic." The twin bases for such a holistic approach lay in humoral theory and in experienced clinicians' empirical observations, which supported the supposition that mind and body functioned as conjoined facets of the whole person. The dearth of sound knowledge of disease mechanisms before the medical advances in the course of the nineteenth century inevitably fostered a reliance on inferences. Medicine was therefore "necessarily" (Rosenberg's word) psychosomatic because it had perforce to draw only on careful attention to readily perceptible symptoms, which, in humoral practice, were directly linked to the patient's disposition and mood.

This prevailing situation of a blend of ignorance and supposition forms the context for the impact of Franz Anton Mesmer (1734–1815). A physician who had completed his medical studies in Vienna in 1766, Mesmer postulated the power of "an imponderable fluid permeating the entire universe, and infusing both matter and spirit with its vital force."[15] He believed that recovery from diseases and disturbances would follow the redistribution of this fluid within the body to achieve equilibrium. This healing process, Mesmer maintained, could be activated with the aid of magnets to draw out the negative qualities of astral and terrestrial fluids. Mesmer presented his system of magnetism as primarily a physical realignment of bodily elements, although skeptics initially gave his therapy the name of "Mesmerism" in order to deny that physical forces were involved. While the genuineness of the trances Mesmer induced was granted, the powers in play remained mysterious, as did the underlying links between mind and body. The treatment in fact relied very heavily on the exercise of interpersonal suggestion; the spellbinding trance evoked by the mesmerist is reminiscent of primitive rites of exorcism. Mesmer sensed the psychological dimensions of many of his patients' illnesses and sought to cure them by psychotherapeutic means in the guise of physical remedies such as magnets, baths, and so on. What is striking about Mesmer is the bizarre combination of practices that smack of magic and charlatanism with his apparently intuitive grasp of the dynamics of psychosomatic disorders.[16]

What then caused the paradigm shift in the course of the nineteenth century that represents so decisive a swing of the pendulum away from the holistic model of the previous centuries? Overall the transformation of medicine can be summarized as a switch from a speculative art (as it was during humoralism) to its modern status as a science. Admittedly, the status of science itself was long unsettled. "Medicine did not simply become more scientific in the nineteenth century," John Harley Warner points out; "what was considered science, and what was not, changed."[17] Issues of power and authority surfaced in the absence of consensus over the meaning and attribution of such words as "expert" and "amateur."[18] Mesmerism offers one salient example of this difficulty in reaching agreement: was it sheer quackery or a scientific procedure (or somewhere in between)?

Still, the nineteenth century made enormous progress in the understanding of the body's physiological and pathological processes. A series of new or improved instruments allowed a deeper probing of the body, giving literally more insight into areas beneath the surface. The first and perhaps most crucial of these instruments was the stethoscope, devised in 1819 by René-Théophile-Hyacinthe Laënnec (1781–1826).[19] Instead of being dependent on patients' subjective narration of their symptoms and on impressionistic surface observations, doctors could by means of the stethoscope arrive at a more objective diagnosis by expert, differentiating interpretation of sounds they themselves heard.

The stethoscope attained its utmost value in combination with the postmortem discoveries in pathological anatomy made by Marie-François-Xavier Bichat (1771–1801). He discovered distinctive lesions in particular organs as the signs of disease. Bichat realized that the source of disease was a *local* abnormality. His findings instigated one of the most fundamental turning-points in the history of medicine: the turn away from patient specificity to disease specificity in diagnosis and therapeutics. Instead of regarding the entire body as being in a state of imbalance, doctors in the wake of Bichat sought to pinpoint the singular lesion at the core of the patient's symptoms. The categoric ravages that Bichat saw in cadavers as the telltale signs of specific diseases could be directly related to the sounds emitted by the living person and picked up by the stethoscope. The connection between what was audible in the patient and what was visible in the cadaver enabled doctors to deduce a firmly grounded diagnostic taxonomy. Each disease—pleurisy, pneumonia, tuberculosis, inflammation of various areas of the heart—was found to have its characteristic sounds in living patients and to be confirmed by the damage revealed in cadavers. The conjunction of pathological anatomy with the stethoscope created a vital link between research and clinical practice and accomplished the transition to the scientific method rooted in pragmatically established facts.

Some fifty years after Bichat, Rudolf Virchow (1821-1902) in his *Cellular Pathology* (1858) engaged in the comparative scrutiny of healthy and diseased tissues. Virchow was literally able to see more exactly than Bichat, following the development of another essential instrument in the meanwhile: the decisive improvement in microscopes beginning in the 1830s and 1840s.[20] So Bichat's gross pathology was succeeded by microscopic pathology, which permitted far greater access to more minute elements of the body.[21] Virchow grasped that how the cell *looks* is only one pointer to the problem; how it *acts* is the crux of its defectiveness.

The scientific character of medicine was also furthered in the 1860s and 1879s by the introduction of the numerical method, the quantification and graphic representation of temperature, pulse and respiration rates. The French researcher Pierre-Charles-Alexandre Louis (1787–1872) championed systematic analysis through statistics on the ground that truth resides in objective facts. If medicine had up to the nineteenth century been "ubiquitously 'psychosomatic,'" it then strove to become progressively more scientific in its thrust to precision.

The increasing number of instruments through which doctors could view internal organs promoted this aim: the urethra-cystic speculum, the laryngoscope, the ophthalmoscope, the endoscope, the bronchoscope all successively took their place in the physician's equipment in the course of the nineteenth century.[22] The century culminated in 1895 in Wilhelm Konrad Röntgen's (1845–1923) X rays, another milestone in medicine's diagnostic armamentarium through visualization. Pathology and instrumentation ushered in "the medicine of the all-powerful gaze."[23]

That gaze was equally decisive in bacteriology in the understanding of germ theory. The meticulous research of the French chemist Louis Pasteur (1822–95) and of the German country doctor Robert Koch (1843–1910) provided convincing proof of the role of microorganisms as the infective agents. Most important, by distinguishing between a spectrum of organisms and isolating the one causing each disease, Pasteur and Koch showed that particular organisms produced specific infections. Their discoveries furthered the localism characteristic of nineteenth-century medicine, the practice of closely examining the diseased part alone, more or less to the exclusion of the rest of the body, let alone patients in their social context. So in the nineteenth century the pendulum swung to a particularism at the opposite pole to the holistic vision of earlier times.

With its emphasis on facts, visible lesions, local sites, and objective truths, the nineteenth century was unlikely to be interested in the shadowlands of psychosomatics. "Ills did not become legitimate until and unless they were somatic," Rosenberg explains, that is, until and unless they could be traced to a specific physical cause.[24] The "aggressively scientist character"[25] of nineteenth-century medical thought was inclined to attribute any failure to reach a physicalist diagnosis to shortcomings in the available instrumentation. "The triumphs celebrated by somatic medicine in the nineteenth century . . . to a very great degree succeeded in wiping out recollection of the attention traditionally accorded to mind-body relationships."[26] Scientific medicine, with its focus on the body, left—or pushed—the mind aside.

So in the course of the nineteenth century the disparity between the progress made in the understanding of the body, on the one hand, and that of the mind, on the other, is glaring. Attempts to gain access to the workings of the mind by scrutiny of the head's surface, such as the facial features in physiognomy and the contours of the skull in phrenology were no more than bogus science. The popularity they enjoyed is a further indication of insecurity about the parameters of science.

Psychiatry declined in esteem through the nineteenth century because of its inability to "clothe the borderland ills . . . in somatic garb,"[27] to identify in the body the precise site of the lesion underlying the aberrant behavior. By contrast, the new discipline of neurology—the study of the brain and the nervous system—rose correspondingly in prestige. Neurologists achieved some important advances in their pursuit of somatic causations. In 1822 Antoine Laurent Bayle (1799–1858), by uncovering the source of the general paralysis of the insane in syphilitic infection, furnished a physical, neurological explanation of what had been taken for a mental disorder.[28] In the 1850s and 1860s Paul Broca (1824–1880) in France and Carl Wernicke (1848–1905) in Germany mapped out areas of brain tissue involved in the formation of words. Shortly thereafter, David Ferrier (1843–1928) in England showed that one discrete part of the monkey's brain was specifically concerned with sensory input. The journal *Brain* was founded in 1866. In 1891 the German Heinrich Wilhelm Waldeyer (1837–1921) posited the neuron theory, according to which the nervous system was not a homogeneous substance but rather a network of separate cells that communicated with one another via long, nearly touching tentacles. The realization that this system was alive with electricity marked a further major step forward.[29] Observation revealed that infectious diseases such as cholera, typhoid fever, or diphtheria could lead to changes in the nervous system and hence to mental symptoms that were somatic in origin. By the 1870s the physical underpinnings of other diseases formerly classified as neuroses had been located: for example, delirium tremens was found to be caused by alcohol, and tetanus by infection in puncture wounds.

So the concept of the lesion gained increasing prominence as the cause of several disorders, previously regarded as mental, was uncovered. Some three hundred autopsies of the brains of epileptics, carried out in France between 1833 and 1854 disclosed almost always a marked divergence in weight between the two hemispheres, indicating a disruption of the normal symmetrical functioning of the two sides of the brain as a source of certain nervous and mental disorders.[30] In 1882 the role of the vasomotor centers of the brain in regulating the dilation and contraction of blood vessels was investigated.[31] Neurology was moving toward the fulfillment of its central purpose of finding scientific explanations for what had hitherto been taken as spiritual, supernatural, or demonic incursions.

Emotional life was thought to be legible in physiological or pathological signs.

Neuropsychiatry thus came more and more to challenge psychiatry, particularly in Germany under the direction of Wilhelm Griesinger (1817–69), who was convinced that mental disorders were brain diseases to be unlocked by neuropathology.[32] While not exclusively a somaticist (he also believed in the pathogenic potential of emotions), Griesinger had a decided physicalist bias that led him to surmount the troubling distinctions between cerebral and mental diseases by according supremacy to the physical. All kinds of organ disturbances, such as spinal irritation, gastric upheavals, blood or vascular abnormalities, local inflammation, adverse bacteria, cerebral cellular alterations, irritation of the mucous membrane, and ovariouterine derangements, were explored with the aim of finding specific bodily causes for mental disorders and thereby transforming what was called "mental physiology" into an exact science. To a period obsessed with the positivistic accumulation of factual knowledge, the quest for lesions was a more legitimate and promising course than the probing of feelings.

Typical of this endeavor to subsume psychological disorders under physiological categories is the notion of "neurasthenia," a term and a malady largely invented by George M. Beard (1839–93). The symptoms of neurasthenia, listed in his medical textbook, *A Practical Treatise on Nervous Exhaustion (Neurasthenia)* (1880), and in the popular version, *American Nervousness: Its Causes and Consequences* (1883), encompass a strange medley of physical and psychological complaints: insomnia, dilated pupils, noises in the ear, muscle spasms, cold feet and hands, dryness of the skin, fear of lightning or of society or of responsibility, dizziness, difficulty in swallowing, gaping and yawning, frequent urination, and so on.[33] Neurasthenia had an "immense capacity to be all things to all medical men"[34] and to all patients. Its very comprehensiveness was a primary attraction to an age that favored a somatic diagnosis, however questionable—and could not always come up with one.[35]

Beard endowed his syndrome with a physicalist basis through the Greek derivation of its name, which gave it a literal meaning of "lack of nerve strength."[36] He drew on the analogy of the electric battery that will give all the light needed when in perfect order with new fluids, clean elements, and good connections, but whose reserves may be so drained as to become "feeble" and "useless."[37] The comparison to such a mechanical system as a battery emphasized the physical nature of neurasthenia. Thus, Margaret Cleaves, an overworked physician in New York City, was told in the later 1880s that she had "sprained [her] brain."[38]

Through his choice of the electric battery as a model, Beard avoided any hint that neurasthenia could have an emotional component, although many of its symptoms strike today's readers as potentially psychosomatic in nature: insomnia, difficulty in swallowing, and dizziness, not to mention such unambiguously psychological disorders as fear of society or responsibility. Beard's neglect, even denial, of feelings exemplifies not only the later nineteenth-century's preference for physicalist diagnoses and treatments but also its determination to separate mind and body.

However, toward the end of the century, the pendulum began to swing back again to a "medicine of the imagination,"[39] partly because neurology was unable to account satisfactorily for a variety of disorders vaguely termed as "nervous" since no pathology was evident.[40] Neurology was more successful in the laboratory than in a clinical setting; its therapeutics lagged far behind its diagnostic capacities, so that disappointment arose at the lack of practical benefits from its scientific discoveries.

Somatic medicine's impotence in the face of certain types of disorder is evidenced in the efforts of the brilliant French neurologist Jean-Martin Charcot (1825–93) to deal with what he called "hysteria." At the Sâlpétrière hospital for women in Paris, Charcot sought to combine pathology with clinical research. In keeping with the trends of the time, he focused on cerebral localization, attempting to determine which parts of the brain or the nervous system were at the root of particular symptoms. But the multifarious manifestations of "hysteria"—paralyses, contractures, muteness, deafness, blindness, fixities—resisted decipherment by neurological means. His ultimate goal was to uncover the underlying lesion, for he presupposed a hidden organicity, although the hospital's microscopic laboratory could not discern any signs of it. In consonance with the somatic view of "hysteria," the remedies applied at La Sâlpétrière were primarily physicalist: compression, friction, massage, electricity, and metallotherapy, the application of copper, silver, or iron bars.[41]

Yet despite his pronounced neurological bent, Charcot did not wholly dismiss psychology, because he noted the effects of the imagination. In commenting on the sudden cure of contracture of a limb in three cases, he does not hesitate to introduce the word: "Chez ces femmes, la guérison était survenue tout d'un coup, au milieu de circonstances bien propres à émouvoir l'imagination"[42] (In these women, the cure occurred all of a sudden under circumstances very apt to affect the imagination). But imagination, along with the entire field of psychology, is appropriated into his theories by translation into physical concepts: "[E]n matière de maladies nerveuses, la psychologie est là, et ce que j'appelle la psychologie, c'est la physiologie rationelle de l'écorce cérébrale"[43] (in nervous diseases, psychology is present, and what I call psychology is the rational physiology of the cerebral cortex). That statement made by Charcot in 1888 explicitly summarizes the later nineteenth-century predilection for subjugating the psychological to the physiological.

Nevertheless, various afflictions continued to defy nineteenth-century somatic medicine. The problem of pain without a diagnosable physical cause became a growing medical and legal issue in the wake of railroad travel and accidents.[44] Various hypotheses were put forward to account for phenomena that contravened medicine's prevailing physicalist orientation. For instance, a pamphlet entitled "The Influence of Railway Travelling on Public Health," published in the *Lancet* in 1862, argued that passengers sustained "a series of small and rapid concussions" (41) from the machinery's vibrations. These suppositions were based on the assumption that shocks could be transmitted from one part of the human being to another. This theory was invoked to explain the cases of passengers who had no ascertainable injuries yet who suffered from such aftereffects of accidents as insomnia or headaches. The inexplicable sequelae of railroad accidents are classic examples of psychosomatic conversion reactions, although this was not understood at the time. Still, physicians concluded that these passengers had been traumatized, and their hurt was becoming manifest in a figurative manner. This conclusion amounted by implication to the concession that mind and body were somehow connected.

How this connection took place was of intense fascination to the British physician Daniel Hack Tuke (1827–95). In his monumental volume *Illustrations of the Influence of the Mind upon the Body in Health and Disease, Designed to Elucidate the Action of the Imagination* (1872) Tuke discusses multiple examples of mystifying bodily manifestations. Although he defines his aim as a "systematic" investigation of cases that puzzled and challenged medical understanding, his work is more speculative than scientific. His basic postulate of the imagination as the operative force immediately removes him from the strictly scientific orbit of experimental medicine. Tuke starts from a fundamental acceptance of a mind-body connection and aims "to ascertain as far as possible "the channels through, and the mode by which this influence is exerted" (x). Bridging psyche and soma, Tuke astutely coins the phrase "psycho-physical phenomena" (xii) for his cases, a phrase that graphically projects the dual involvement of mind and body in their formation.

Tuke shows a genuine appreciation of "the profound influence of the Mind upon the Body" (xii) by positing that feelings such as fear, anxiety, fright, anger, disappointed ambition, grief, or joy can precipitate a physical response. He cites a variety of examples of such interaction: A twenty-year-old woman, on seeing a mouse running under a table at the other end of the room, "uttered an exclamation of alarm, and in an instant entirely lost the power of audible speech" (254). Another woman, after seeing one of her children scald herself and rescuing her, falls into a catatonic state that still persists three weeks after her admission to hospital (255). An eight-year-old girl, separated from her mother, exhibits delirium, headaches, and an inability to stand, all resistant to every form of treatment, but recovers spontaneously when she is reunited with her mother (259–60). All these cases are patently psychosomatic in character.

But when Tuke moves from illustration to tentative explanations, he falls back upon the accepted somatic concepts of medical reasoning. His hypotheses devolve as much from reference to physiological as to psychological processes. For example, in considering paralysis as a result of loss of muscular power, Tuke comments "that the motor centres are frequently enfeebled by the abnormal play of emotion upon them," yet adds at once that "an emotion may also be conceived to cause a structural change in the higher centres of the encephalon." He concludes that it is "sudden vascular changes in the brain which interfere with its nutrition," thereby causing paralysis "directly, through the direct nerve channels, and indirectly, through the vaso-motor nerves" (246). Spasms, contractions, "nerve energy" (356—Beard's favorite formulation), "cerebral ischemia" (258)—this is the physicalist terminology that Tuke chooses. The idea of the imagination proves inadequate as a usable key to the psychosomatic disorders of which Tuke was certainly aware. Ultimately, therefore, his *Influence of the Mind upon the Body* is most interesting for the delicate balance between the insights it offers and the limitations it reveals in the understanding of psychological mechanisms at that time.[45] The swing of the pendulum back toward the psychological in the later nineteenth century was for long impeded by both the dominance of somatic medicine and the lack of a cogent framework for the interpretation of "psycho-physical phenomena."

That framework was delineated only at the turn of the century in Freud's *Studies on Hysteria* (1895), *Interpretation of Dreams* (1900), and in the case history known as "Dora" (1905).[46] Like Charcot and Tuke, Freud was trained as a neurologist and achieved recognition early in his life for his research in that field. He was in fact perturbed by the direction his work took when he relinquished neuroscience in favor of psychology. Freud's unease at this juncture of his career shows how he himself had been conditioned to value scientific medicine more highly than the then decidedly less rigorous and even somewhat dubious realm of psychology. But his clinical experiences with his patients convinced him that the standard repertoire of treatments of the day—rest, hydrotherapy, electrotherapy, massage—were ineffective in curing "nervous" diseases. It was in the course of Freud's daily massage of Emmy von N . . . , the first case reported in the *Studies on Hysteria,* that she began to talk as if casually, producing each time the memories and associations that had occurred to her since their previous conversation. When Freud realized that her talk was by no means as unintentional ("absichtslos")[47] or casual as it seemed, he hit upon the strategy of free association, the cornerstone of psychoanalysis.

Through patients' spontaneous talk Freud came to intuit the existence of a subconscious layer of the mind that unwittingly determines behavior and that may surface in ways both unexpected and uncontrolled by the conscious mind, such as slips of the tongue, forgetting, or speaking obliquely through the body. The concept of the unconscious,[48] so conspicuously absent from Tuke's work, represents an enormous advance on mere "imagination." By surmising the power of the unconscious, Freud was able to suggest the mechanisms whereby "psycho-physical" or psychosomatic disorders become manifest. He projected the mind as layered into three discrete but communicating levels: the id, the ego, and the superego. This conceptualization led Freud to a frequent use of images drawn from archeology, as though the mind were organized like a site to be excavated. The theory that he formulated of the influence of the mind on the body is thus essentially psychological. Much later, in his monograph *Das Ich und das Es* (1923; *The Ego and the Id*), he endorsed the view of the writer-psychoanalyst Georg Groddeck, "dass wir . . . 'gelebt' werden von unbekannten, unbeherrschbaren Mächten" (that we are "lived" by unknown, uncontrollable powers).[49] Given Freud's stylistic precision, his adoption of the passive form ("lived by") must be read as a particularly emphatic and revealing turn of phrase.

Freud's perspicacious understanding of the role of the unconscious in our daily behavior has been hailed as "the magic key"[50] to the mind-body problem. This claim, put forward by Felix Deutsch, who was associated with Freud, is perhaps something of an overstatement, since even now that problem has not been wholly solved. However, the recognition of the vital significance of the unconscious in the history of psychosomatic medicine can hardly be sufficiently underscored. The elaboration of psychoanalysis marks the crucial turning point in the return swing of the pendulum away from the wholehearted privileging of the somatic prevalent in the mid- to later nineteenth century. By positing an unremitting and often decisive input from the unconscious mind into our manifest conduct in health and in illness, psychoanalysis renewed the link between psyche and soma.

While the importance of psychoanalysis for the rehabilitation of the holistic approach of psychosomatic medicine is beyond question, Freud's contribution to psychosomatics has tended to be underestimated. Paul Roazen, for instance, asserts that "Freud had only a slight interest" in the field of psychosomatics,[51] while Lipowski points out that "Freud used the term 'conversion' to refer to the process whereby psychic excitation was transmuted into somatic symptoms, but he confined his hypothesis to hysteria."[52] This comment overlooks the fact that in the early years of psychoanalysis, still following nineteenth-century usage, "hysteria" was the normative term, which was only gradually superseded (largely due to Freud's work) by "neurosis" or "psychoneurosis." The allegation that "Freud had only a slight interest" in psychosomatics is conclusively refuted by Deutsch's and Elvin V. Semrad's "Survey of Freud's Writings on the Conversion Symptom,"[53] which documents his continuing concern with the phenomenon of conversion from 1894 right up to 1938, the year before his death.

The underestimation of Freud's interest in psychosomatic disorders was likely fostered by the fact that he published just one article overtly devoted to a psychosomatic conversion: "Die psychogene Sehstörung in psychoanalytischer Auffassung" (1910; "Psychogenic Visual Disturbances According to Psychoanalytic Conceptions"). Taking inexplicable blindness as the prototype of a psychogenic disturbance, Freud argues that it is the product of "Auto-suggestion" (95 [105]). How this may occur, he goes on, is incomprehensible "ohne den Begriff des 'Unbewussten' zu Hilfe zu nehmen" (95; "without recourse to the concept of 'the unconscious'" [106]). A condition such as functional blindness is the outcome not just of dissociation but of a fundamentally dynamic "Spiel von einander fördernden und hemmenden Kräften" (96; "interplay of reciprocally urging and checking forces" [107]).

Freud proposes the term "Verdrängung" ("repression") for this process. While repression is the accepted translation for "Verdrängung" in psychology, the literal meaning of the German word is to supplant. The difference between the customary and the literal translation is important. "To repress" denotes to keep down, restrain, curb, check, overcome; "to supplant" means to take the place of, oust, usurp a position or function. This dual signification is particularly apposite to psychosomatic disorders in which emotions are simultaneously kept down and displaced into the body. What is more, the root of "Verdrängung" is "Drang" (urge, drive). It is, Freud adds, "das Misslingen der Verdrängung" (97; "miscarriages of repression" [108]) that are the fundamental cause of symptom formation. When repression is not fully accomplished, conversion sets in as the feelings, which the patient wishes to banish but cannot do so entirely, speak through the body, for example in blindness. Eloquently Freud concludes that conversion represents "die Rache, die Entschädigung des verdrängten Triebes" (99; "the revenge, the indemnification of the repressed impulse" [110]). He cites further examples of the intricate relation of organs to the conscious ego, on the one hand, and to repression, on the other, noting with an insight based on his extensive clinical experience that it is the motor organs that are most liable to be affected. Thus the hand that had desired to commit an act of sexual aggression becomes hysterically crippled after the inhibition of this desire and can do nothing else; similarly, the fingers of those who have renounced masturbation refuse to acquire the delicate mobility required for the piano or violin (100; [110–11]).[54]

What Freud designates in the closing words of that article as the "'somatisches Entgegenkommen' des Organs" (102 "'somatic compliance' of the organs" [112]) is consistently illustrated in the *Studies on Hysteria*, where each of the patients presents with one or more physical complaints. It is essential to remember that in consulting Freud they were all going to a neurologist (not a psychiatrist) in the firm belief that their symptoms were somatic. Emmy von N . . . suffers from insomnia, stomach pains, fear of animals, sporadic bouts of stammering, diffuse aches and pains, sundry tics, capriciousness in eating, and a refusal to drink water. Lucy R . . . is dogged by a persistent smell of burnt pudding and later of smoking. Katharina is beset by attacks exhibiting palpitations, shortness of breath, hammering in her head, a sense of choking, pressure on her eyes, fear, and visions of a terrifying face. Elisabeth von R . . . has for two years had pain in her legs that impedes her mobility. In each of these cases the patient is relieved of her symptomatology by Freud's eliciting the story of its hidden etiology.

The idea of conversion, as Deutsch's and Semrad's survey shows, is pivotal to Freud's theories. Freud repeatedly uses the term *Konversion* throughout the *Studies on Hysteria*, defining it with characteristic clarity and precision: "anstatt der seelischen Schmerzen, die sie sich erspart hatte, traten körperliche auf"[55] (in place of spiritual pain which she [Elisabeth] spared herself, physical pain appeared). The effects of conversion are striking too in a further subsidiary case introduced parenthetically in the *Studies on Hysteria,* that of Cäcilie, who had for fifteen years suffered violent attacks of facial neuralgia that occured two or three times a year and lasted five to six days. The pain was resistant to all the then normative modes of treatment, such as electrotherapy, locally applied medications, and laxatives(!). In an intervention reminiscent of the many surgeries some of Barbour's patients had undergone, Cäcilie had even had seven teeth extracted, to no avail. Under growing doubts as to the source of this implacable neuralgia, and curious whether a psychological cause could be unveiled, Freud evokes "die Reproduktion des traumatischen Erlebnisses"[56] (the reproduction of the traumatic experience). The scene that Cäcilie recalls provides the key to her affliction: she had experienced a deep hurt inflicted by a comment of her husband's "wie ein Schlag ins Gesicht"[57] (like a slap in the face). The psychological injury comes to be supplanted and symbolized by, that is, converted into a recurrent bodily torment.

Insistence on "somatic compliance" is central to the case of Dora too, where exactly the same phraseology occurs as in the article on psychogenic blindness: "ein gewisses somatisches Entgegenkommen."[58] The German term "Entgegenkommen" is particularly illuminating: literally, a certain somatic coming-toward, a confluence of the physical symptom and its psychological origin. Freud emphasizes both the reciprocity of body and mind and the absolute necessity for "eine psychische Bedeutung, einen *Sinn*" ("a psychical significance, a *meaning*")[59] to underpin and sustain the symptom. Throughout his reflections on the interpretation of the materials in this complicated case, Freud has repeated recourse to concepts fundamental to psychosomatic medicine: "Konversion" (conversion), which he defines as "die Ubertragung der rein psychischen Bewegung ins Körperliche" ("the translation of a purely psychical excitation into physical terms")[60] "Verdrängung" ("repression," "supplanting") and "Verschiebung" ("displacement). In these latter words, the German particle "Ver-" conveys the sense of something gone askew, pushed or shoved out of its proper place, as happens when the psyche speaks through the body.

Freud's work is the major landmark in the return swing of the pendulum away from the fragmentation resulting from nineteenth-century localistic medicine to the recovery of a more holistic model in a number of ways: in the primary function he accorded to the unconscious in motivation, in his clear perception of physical complaints as expressions of a psychological malaise, and not least in his outspoken championship of the need to take a more comprehensive view of the patient. He argues that the nature of the facts that form the material of psychoanalysis oblige analysts to pay as much attention in their case histories to the purely human and social circumstances of their patients as to the somatic data and the symptoms of the disorder.[61]

The imperative of heeding "the purely human and social circumstances of our patients" in the course of psychoanalysis is a clear precedent to Engel's plea for the biopsychosocial approach. Although psychoanalysis had rather gone out of fashion by the time that Engel put forward his model of patient care, it nonetheless represents a potent paradigm for the perception of the sick person not only as an inseparable entity of mind and body but also as a human being often affected by environmental circumstances and social pressures. Psychoanalysis marks a more modern reprise of an approach that is, like pre-nineteenth-century medicine, "necessarily and ubiquitously 'psychosomatic.'"

CHAPTER THREE

The Mysterious Leap

Only connect.
—E. M. Forster,
A Passage to India

"**M**ysterious" or "puzzling"? These are two possible translations of the word Freud applied to what he called the leap from the mind to the body typical of psychosomatic conversion disorders. His own phrase in the seventeenth lecture of the *Vorlesungen zur Einführung in die Psychoanalyse* (1916–17) is "jener rätselhafter Sprung aus dem Seelischen ins Körperliche" (that puzzling leap from the soul to the body).[1] In the American translation, titled *A General Introduction to Psychoanalysis* (1920), the unnamed translator has opted for "that mysterious leap from the psyche to the physical."[2] Freud's word, derived from the common German word "Rätsel" (puzzle, riddle) suggests something amenable ultimately to solution, whereas "mysterious" points more toward the metaphysical realm of insoluble enigmas, except in its popular usage of the mysteries in detective fiction that are disentangled by a clever sleuth. Perhaps the difference between "puzzling" and "mysterious" reflects either a more or a less optimistic view of the likelihood of an eventual deciphering of the mechanisms of conversion. With a remarkable prescience that foresaw the evolution of psychiatry in the twentieth century from psychoanalysis to psychoneuroimmunology, Freud is reported to have stated during one of the last scientific meetings at his house "that he had to hurry up, because 'endocrinology' was already at the heels of analysis."[3]

That pronouncement is cited in the book that naturalized Freud's phrase in the United States: *The Mysterious Leap from the Mind to the Body* (1959). Its editor and primary contributor, Felix Deutsch, who had for a while been Freud's personal physician in Vienna, emigrated in 1934 to Boston, where he founded the Psychoanalytic Institute. Deutsch's extensive

37

early experience in internal medicine coalesced with his subsequent interest in psychoanalysis to provide excellent preparation for his concentration on psychosomatics.

The first part of *The Mysterious Leap* is devoted to the phrase and the topic of conversion, notably in the section "Is the Term 'Mysterious Leap' Warranted?" (11–26). The eleven discussants, all physicians, express a variety of opinions, some welcoming the designation, while others voice reservations. The most stimulating comment, certainly from the humanistic angle, is the affirmation of the phrase as "a metaphor" that helps "to bring order into experience" (18). Deutsch insists that Freud did not think in terms of "a dichotomy or a dualism" but that "he considered the transition from a psychic process into a bodily symptom enigmatic" (vii).

"Enigmatic," "mysterious," and "puzzling" it has continued to be throughout the medical literature of the twentieth century. The focus of the debates, along with their terminology, has undergone successive modifications over the decades with the shift from a predominantly psychological to the recent increasing emphasis on the biochemical factors that control the mind. The term "psychosomatic" itself has been subject less to attack than to dismissal. In the American Psychiatric Association's official *Diagnostic and Statistical Manual* it has been consistently avoided and replaced since the 1980 edition by "somatoform." Richard Halgin and Susan Whitbourne assert that the word "has been abandoned because it acquired a popular meaning that suggested that such physical problems are 'in the person's head.'"[4] Nevertheless, "psychosomatic" has remained in currency: despite talk of the possibility of a name change, the professional group in the field continues to call itself the American Psychosomatic Society.

This verbal vagrancy serves as a constant reminder of the essential elusiveness of the disorders with which it is concerned, as well as of the continuing disagreements among practitioners wrestling with the phenomenon. The shifts of opinion are not as radical as the swings of the pendulum in the nineteenth century, but the repeated revisions show the struggles involved in the many attempts to attain a firmer grasp of the nature of that mysterious leap.

Deutsch was among the influx of psychoanalysts and analytically oriented physicians into the United States following the rise of Nazism, which gave a potent impetus not only to the growth of psychoanalysis in the United States but also to a renewal of the awareness of psychosomatic elements in some illnesses. According to Rosenberg, somatic medicine had established such supremacy in this country in the first decades of the twentieth century that "it is not surprising that the term *psychosomatic* and the interests it stood for could in fact seem novel and reformist in the late 1930s and 1940s."[5] The crux of that novelty and reform lay less in the actual techniques of psychoanalysis than in the recognition of the reciprocal interdependence of mind and body.

The word "emotion" opens the title of the landmark volume that inaugurated the synoptic study of psychosomatics, *Emotions and Bodily Changes: A Survey of Literature on Psychosomatic Interrelationships, 1910–1933,* by Dunbar. Published in 1935 and revised in 1938, it is "essentially a bibliography" (xiv), a compilation of abstracts intended as a foundation for further research. The detailed review of the professional literature in the extensive bibliography (435–566), which comprises 2,358 entries, is arranged by organ groups: the nervous system, musculature, endocrines, general metabolism, heat regulation, the cardiovascular system, the respiratory system including otorhinolaryngology, the gastrointestinal system, the genitourinary system and gynecology, the special sense systems, and the skin. In each of these areas, Dunbar underscores the cardinal significance of the emotions in the genesis and development of disorders: "Scientific study of the emotions and of the bodily changes that accompany diverse emotional experience marks a new era in medicine. . . . We lack perspective concerning our knowledge in this field and are confused in our concepts of the interrelationship of psychic, including emotional, and somatic processes in health and disease" (xi). Dunbar exhorts physicians to pay greater attention to the role of emotions in order to attain a "total picture" of the patient (66). This stance represents vigorous support for the holism that is one of the fundamental principles of psychosomatic medicine.

Balancing her crusading spirit with prudence, Dunbar endorses the coexistence of "a somatic as well as a psychic component in every disease" (67). She outspokenly condemns the alternative of "physical or psychic" in favor of the subtler question: "To what extent is the disease physical and to what extent psychic?" (428). She urges the combination of twentieth-century diagnostic and therapeutic methods with a pretechnological holistic assessment of the patient because the parts and the whole are inextricably linked and can only be understood as a unified entity. Without using the more modern term "biopsychosocial," Dunbar foreshadows its thrust toward comprehensiveness and an appreciation of complexity. The adjective she chooses is "stereoscopic," which she defines as "the study of simultaneous sequences in psychic and somatic spheres" (xxi), that is, two pictures of the same object from slightly different points of view (in photography corresponding to the position of the two eyes) and united into a single image. Dunbar's essentially monistic perception of body and mind as a unified entity leads her to document interconnectedness rather than to probe the mysteries of the leap.

Dunbar's *Emotions and Bodily Changes* marks the beginning of a new phase in the study of psychosomatics. In 1938 the Tenth International Congress for Psychotherapy devoted a major section to psychosomatic problems, as did the Association for Research in Nervous and Mental Disease later that year. The journal *Psychosomatic Medicine* was founded in 1939. Its introductory statement specifies that "its object is to study in their interrelation the psychological and physiological aspects of all normal and abnormal bodily functions and thus to integrate somatic therapy and psychotherapy."[6]

Such integration of somatic therapy and psychotherapy is also the purpose of Dunbar's second book, *Psychosomatic Diagnosis* (1943; 2d ed., 1948). A 741-page textbook, it is designed primarily to teach interviewing methods that would elicit the patient's psychological profile together with the physical history. Dunbar recommends the use of open, inviting questions along with a stance on the doctor's part conducive to the patient's relaxation. As in *Emotions and Bodily Changes* she dwells on the basic imperative of "both/and" not "either/or" thinking (6) so as to bear in mind the "continuous interplay between emotion and physiology" (8). The year 1943 also saw the appearance of another textbook in the field, *Psychosomatic Medicine: The Clinical Application of Psychopathology to General Medical Problems* by Edward Weiss and O. Spurgeon English.

Dunbar's successors in the early 1950s were more directly influenced by Freud than she was. Foremost among them was Franz Alexander (1891–1964), who was considered one of Freud's best pupils.[7] After a period in the late 1920s in Berlin, then one of the main centers of psychoanalysis, Alexander emigrated to the United States, where he founded the Chicago Institute for Psychoanalysis in 1932. A leader in psychosomatic medicine, he made a significant impact on clinical practice by drawing attention to the effect of specific psychic conflicts on certain types of disorders.[8]

Alexander's major work, *Psychosomatic Medicine: Its Principles and Applications* (1950), follows on his earlier book on the medical value of psychoanalysis. Alexander's firm allegiance to the psychoanalytic approach is evident from the outset. He begins by attacking "the 'dual personality' of the modern clinician" who assumes "a 'scientific' attitude which is essentially only a dogmatic antipsychological attitude" (23). In rebuttal, Alexander categorically affirms the importance of psychoanalysis for the development of medicine (24–34). His rootedness in psychoanalysis is also amply demonstrated in his terminology: he writes of "psychoneuroses," of "gastric neuroses," which are "responses to emotional stress" that "can best be described as 'regressive patterns' because they represent a revival of bodily responses to emotional tensions which are characteristic of the infant" (63). The quotation marks surrounding 'regressive patterns' denote a reference back to Freud. In keeping with his allegiance to psychoanalysis, Alexander believes that "the mind rules the body," and that this is "the most fundamental fact which we know about the process of life" (37). For this reason he postulates "that the psychological factors influencing physiological processes must be subjected to the same detailed and careful scrutiny as is customary in the study of physiological processes" (11). In the wake of Freud, he defines a conversion symptom as "a *symbolic* expression of an emotionally charged psychological content: it is an attempt to discharge the emotional tension" (42).

Alexander, even more so than Dunbar, constantly underscores the patient's fundamental wholeness as an integrated entity. The patient is "a human being with worries, fears, hopes, and despairs . . . and not merely the bearer of organs—of a diseased liver or stomach" (17). Repeatedly he insists that "the patient's problems cannot be divided into physical and mental; they must be treated in their totality" (270). For "psychological and somatic phenomena take place in the same organism and are merely two aspects of the same process" (52). Therefore "psychosomatic" does not imply "a dichotomy between mind and body"; on the contrary, "this dichotomy is precisely what the psychosomatic point of view tries to avoid" (49) through "the simultaneous and co-ordinated use of somatic—i.e., physiological, anatomical, pharmacological, surgical, and dietary—methods and concepts on the one hand, and psychological methods and concepts on the other" (50). Thus "the psychosomatic approach is a multidisciplinary procedure in which psychiatrists collaborate with experts in the different branches of medicine" (13).

Alexander's comprehensive perception of the patient leads directly to his insistence on the incorporation of the social dimension. He sees "the continuous functional stress arising during the everyday life of the individual . . . in our contact with the environment" (47–48) as a major source of illness. This conviction clearly derives from the practice in psychoanalysis of relating patient to environment, particularly to family, as the locus of many tensions and conflicts. In this insight Alexander anticipates Engel's biopsychosocial model by some thirty years. Alexander posits a mysterious interconnectedness between all facets of the patient's being rather than a mysterious leap from mind to body.

The expansiveness of Alexander's vision underlies his theory of the multicausality of all disease. Immunological vulnerability, emotional elements, and social stressors interact with each other in the etiology and maintenance of disease. Often Alexander seems intent on subsuming all disease into the category for which he is spokesman, as in his claim that "[t]heoretically every disease is psychosomatic" (52). But such sweeping assertions have to be read as part of Alexander's belief that "emotional factors influence all bodily processes through nervous and humoral pathways" (52). They also need to be seen in the context of the increasing fragmentation of somatic medicine at that time. As early as 1927 Frances W. Peabody, in one of a series of lectures delivered at Harvard Medical School, issued the warning that "the institutional eye tends to become focused on the lung, and it forgets that the lung is only one member of the body."[9]

The ulterior problem inherent in Alexander's *Psychosomatic Medicine* stems from the kind of leveling that his conviction of the ubiquity of the psychosomatic entails. Like Dunbar, Alexander surveys "Emotional Factors in Different Diseases" (part 2, 83–215), identifying certain diseases, notably asthma, gastric ulcer, ulcerative colitis, and dermatitis, as primary manifestations of the likely effects of emotional factors on the origins and course of disease. But he minimizes, even repudiates, any basic distinction between purely somatic and psychosomatic afflictions as a result of his belief that emotional factors are involved in *every* disease. Alexander brushes away the gradations: "[P]sychological processes are fundamentally not different from other processes which take place in the organism. They are at the same time physiological processes and differ from other bodily processes only in that they are perceived subjectively and can be communicated to others verbally" (11). Yet in the very passage in which he argues against differences between psychological and other body processes, Alexander ironically ends by actually naming a cardinal difference: that "psychological processes can be communicated verbally to others." In psychosomatic disorders, in lieu of speech, the communication is mediated through the body, which becomes the carrier of the unvoiced distress. In this bypassing of the normative channels of communication in favor of other paths lies the essence of that mysterious leap which Alexander pushes aside through his emphasis on the seamless cohesiveness of mind and body.

Alexander is the preeminent exponent of psychosomatic medicine precisely because he presses monism to its utmost possibility. By placing psychological and physiological processes on the same level he seeks to demystify, but he can do so only at the expense of underrating the importance of the patient's ability to speak out and the consequent repression that are at the core of psychosomatic conversion. While Alexander provides powerful evidence of the incidence of the leap from mind to body, he shows far less interest in probing how it occurs. Perhaps because he was writing in the fairly early phase of psychosomatic medicine in the twentieth century, he is more concerned to prove the reality of the leap than to investigate the mystery of its hidden processes.

In the half century following the work of Alexander, paramount changes have taken place in the perception of psychosomatic disorders. Nowhere is the development more clearly illustrated than in the successive editions of the American Psychiatric Association's *Diagnostic and Statistical Manual* (*DSM*) from volume 1 (1952) through volume 4 (1994).

The most striking feature of these volumes is the absence of the term "psychosomatic" itself, except in one instance where the reason for its rejection is given (*DSM-I*, 29). This does not mean a lack of attention to this entire area, only the choice of a series of alternative terminologies in the various editions. The volumes' formulations, including the avoidance of "psychosomatic," are determined by their primary aim of acting as a reliable tool for differential diagnosis. They are, therefore, and increasingly so in the two most recent versions, as far as possible factually descriptive, delimiting, and exclusionary. They seek to establish the characteristic features of and distinctions between various mental and emotional disorders for clinical practice. Causation and origins are not central to such an endeavor. However, psychosomatic disturbances demand precisely the type of psychodynamic investigation of their etiology favored by psychoanalysis but not germane to the intentions of the *DSM*, whose precedent is Emil Kraepelin's classificatory *Compendium* (1889).

The first two editions (*DSM-I* [1952]) and *DSM-II* [1968]) show pronounced similarities, both in their relative brevity (130 and 134 pages respectively) and in the philosophy that shapes their terminology. In proposing the class of "Psychophysiologic Autonomic and Visceral Disorders," *DSM-I* explains this verbal usage on the following grounds: "This term is used in preference to 'psychosomatic disorders,' since the latter term refers to a point of view on the discipline of medicine as a whole rather than to certain specified conditions" (29). A so-called psychophysiological reaction is regarded as "the visceral expression of affect which may be thereby largely prevented from being conscious" (29). The undertow of Freudian thought is apparent in the perception of the psychophysiologic manifestation as a substitute outlet for unconscious feelings, although the symptoms are viewed as physiological rather than symbolizing. Such psychosphysiological reactions are then arranged in *DSM-I*, as in Dunbar and Alexander, according to the diverse organ systems, that is, skin, musculoskeletal, respiratory, cardiovascular, hemic and lymphatic, gastrointestinal, genitourinary, endocrine, nervous system (including general fatigue and what was "formerly called 'neurasthenia'" [31]).

In every instance the distinctive feature resides in the determination that "emotional factors are found to play a causative role" (30 and 31, passim). This represents the belief that psychosomatic disorders are essentially psychogenic in origin. A category parallel to "psychophysiological" though more intense, "Psychoneurotic Disorders," obviously Freudian in derivation, covers conversion reactions, which were subsequently designated as a major psychosomatic form. A psychoneurotic disorder arises from anxiety that is "'converted' into functional symptoms in organs or parts of the body, usually those that are mainly under voluntary control" (32–33). The need for quotation marks around "converted" is a telling indication of the novelty, or at least unfamiliarity, of the concept at that time.

DSM-II (1968) is largely a reiteration of its predecessor, with the notable exception that the term "reaction" is dropped. Likewise proclaiming itself as "Prepared by the Committee on Nomenclature and Statistics" to formulate widely valid classificatory codes, it adopts the same descriptive phrase, "Psychophysiologic Disorders," which it defines as "physical disorders of presumably psychogenic origin" (46). The relevant section is rather shorter than that in *DSM-I*. Greater attention is paid in *DSM-II* to the various "Neuroses" (39–41), one of which is designated as "Hysterical neurosis, conversion type," which "must be distinguished from psychophysiologic disorders, which are mediated by the autonomic nervous system" (40). The few departures from *DSM-I*, for instance the description of neurasthenia as a "neurasthenic neurosis" (40), are deliberately underscored, but the similarity of *DSM-II* to *DSM-I* is far greater than the differences between them. Neither comes to incisive grips with the phenomenon of the psychosomatic; only the causative role of emotional factors in a large spectrum of physical disturbances is affirmed.

A radical transformation occurs with *DSM-III* (1980), which, at 496 pages, is more than three times as long as *DSM-II*. This sudden enormous expansion was motivated by the desire for ever more exact differential diagnoses. So the number of discrete disorders rose from 180 in *DSM-II* to 265 in *DSM-III* (and 294 in *DSM-IV*). Each disorder had to meet several stringent criteria in order to conform to a diagnostic code. The overall effect of this nosological rigor was to produce "a science-driven document,"[10] one "decked out with the accouterments of scientific research."[11] The word "accouterments" is slightly derogatory in suggesting the trappings of scientific research rather than much substance. However, advances in the understanding of brain chemistry as well as the introduction of more and more psychotropic drugs were undoubtedly crucial in impelling *DSM-III* toward biological psychiatry.

Political forces were equally decisive in the reshaping of the entire volume. Historians of psychiatry have given vivid accounts of the conflicts and polemics among the members of the coordinating committee.[12] In addition to internal clashes, pressures were exerted by such external groups as gays and lesbians, feminists, and Vietnam War veterans, not to mention insurance companies. But the bone of contention was the position of psychoanalysis, whose prestige had been declining as that of psychopharmacology was rising. Whereas almost a third of the members on the committee for *DSM-I* belonged to psychoanalytic organizations or can be deemed sympathetic to psychoanalysis on the basis of their writings, the committee in charge of *DSM-III* was weighted against psychoanalysis. Its chairman, Dr. Robert Spitzer of Columbia University, though himself trained as an analyst, favored by the 1970s a pattern of diagnosis that corresponded as nearly as possible to observable behaviors rather than to a priori theories that had come to seem questionable to many clinicians. Thus in both *DSM III* and *IV* "psychological factors were assigned to a secondary role as merely ancillary elements," whereas "the earlier definitions carried the implication that psychological factors played an important etiological role in the production of bodily symptoms."[13] This shift of focus from a psychosocial model to a research-based medical one was unpropitious for psychosomatic disturbances, which have proven more open to interpretation from a psychosocial than from a strictly medicalized angle.

The new philosophy is readily apparent in the terminology of *DSM-III*. The cumbersome "psychophysiological" of *DSM-I* and *II* is replaced by the crisper "somatoform." The word "somatoform" itself denotes a reversal of the priorities projected by "psychophysiologic": the earlier formulation posits the primacy of the psyche manifesting itself in the physiological, in contrast to "somatoform," which places the body in the forefront as the site of the disorder. Like somatic medicine, psychiatry now begins with the concrete presenting symptoms. The importance of the Freudian unconscious and of emotions is thereby considerably attenuated, though not completely banished, as the opening definition shows: "The essential features of this group of disorders are symptoms suggesting physical disorder (hence, Somatoform) for which there are no demonstrable organic findings or known physiological mechanisms and for which there is positive evidence, or a strong presumption, that the symptoms are linked to psychological factors or conflicts" (241). The style of reasoning is clearly allied to the medical methodology of ruling out: "Although the symptoms of Somatoform Disorders are 'physical,' the specific pathophysiological processes involved are not demonstrable or understandable by existing laboratory procedures and are conceptualized most clearly using psychological constructs" (241). In these definitions, such phrases as "positive evidence" and "demonstrable or understandable by existing laboratory procedures" point to the adoption of the mentality and methods of somatic medicine. The conceptualization by means of "psychological constructs" seems to come almost as an afterthought; the psychological origins of somatoform disorders are only "a strong presumption" because there is "apparently" (241) no ascertainable physical causation. Caution is here on the verge of intensification into skepticism.

Four types of somatoform disorder are listed in *DSM-III*. "Somatization Disorder," the most common and chronically polysymptomatic, replaces what had previously been known as hysteria. "Conversion Disorder" supersedes "Hysterical Neurosis, Conversion Type" (which is still included, albeit in parentheses). "Psychogenic Pain Disorder" is the third category, while the fourth is an amorphous ("residual") "Atypical Somatoform Disorder." For each type the distinctive diagnostic criteria are laid down together with the characteristic "associated features," such as age of onset, gender ratio, predisposing factors, course, prevalence, familial patterns, impairments and complications. Besides its aspiration to precise diagnoses, *DSM-III* is conspicuous for its elimination of such Freudian concepts and terms as "hysteria" and "psychoneurosis," and, as a consequence, for its determination to remove "*physical disorders in which psychological factors often play an important role, such as irritable colon or bronchial asthma*" (246; note the emphasis) from the psychiatric into the medical realm. As a combined result of these reformulations, the catchment for the elusive psychosomatic disorders was vastly reduced.

DSM-IV (1994) follows the path of *DSM-III* in nosology and terminology, taking them even further along the same lines. Its length, at a hefty 886 pages, is nearly double that of *DSM-III*. By and large, in language more direct than that of its immediate antecedent, its goal is ever greater differentiation between syndromes, so that it at once proliferates more discrete disorders and establishes further exclusionary criteria. The opening of the section on Somatoform Disorders is more straightforward in its wording: "The common feature of the Somatoform Disorders is the presence of physical symptoms that suggest a general medical condition (hence, the term *somatoform*) and are not fully explained by a general medical condition, by the direct effects of a substance, or by another mental disorder" (445). To this category two new subheadings are added: "Undifferentiated Somatoform Disorder," "characterized by unexplained physical complaints lasting at least 6 months, that are below the threshold for a diagnosis of Somatization Disorder" (445), and "Body Dysmorphic Disorder," "the preoccupation with an imagined or exaggerated defect in physical appearance" (445). An explicit distinction is now also drawn between somatoform disorders and "Psychological Factors Affecting Medical Conditions." This amounts to the tacit recognition that many medical conditions are affected by psychological factors, but these are now excluded from the realm of the psychosomatic. Only where no organic pathology is ascertainable is the somatoform diagnosis applicable. This strict limitation is forcefully brought out at the close of the opening paragraph on somatoform disorders: "The grouping of these disorders in a single section is based on clinical utility (i.e., the need to exclude occult general medical conditions or substance-induced etiologies for the bodily symptoms) rather than on assumptions regarding shared etiology or mechanism" (445). Still, *DSM-IV* takes care to warn that "the onset of multiple physical symptoms late in life is almost always due to a general medical condition" (448). The possibility of a latent organic disease in its early stages before it has crystallized into a recognizable syndrome must be weighed against the presence of a psychosomatic disorder. This caveat is another indirect reminder that the divide between functional and organic is more fluid than is generally supposed.

The cumulative impact of the successive editions of *DSM* has been to reduce the arena of the psychosomatic by circumscribing it with growing severity. One important factor in this change is the introduction of several generations of effective psychotropic drugs, which have moved psychiatry away from the "just talk"[14] of psychotherapy toward psychopharmacology, which can in many cases achieve speedier results (and at less cost). The extent to which psychosomatic disorders respond to drugs remains an open question.

DSM-IV has been called "the Bible of Psychiatry"[15] (in a negative sense) because of its stranglehold on the profession through its establishment of universally recognized diagnostic categories. The accusation that it has led to "Pathologizing Everyday Life"[16] is less telling than other possible criticisms. It has repositioned psychiatry away from a humanistic, individual-centered view to a behavioristic methodology that brings it into line with mainstream somatic medicine. Whether this change is welcome is a matter of fundamental dispute in the psychiatric community.[17] The attempted analogy with physical disorders has encouraged an emphasis on overt behaviors, biochemical markers, and cognitive deficits, an objectifying factuality that has as its corollary the displacement of emotions from the core of psychiatry.

This shift of concentration onto a research-based medical model with its focus on brain chemistry is detrimental to the study of psychosomatic disorders as they are not primarily biochemical in etiology. Because the patient's past experiences and social environment are of such vital importance in these disorders, they are far more amenable to a psychodynamic approach. The role of "severe psychosocial stress as a predisposing factor" is still mentioned in *DSM-III* (248), but by *DSM-IV* there is greater emphasis on "Recording Procedures" and "Associated Laboratory Findings," if any (459) than on feelings. Psychology has been supplanted as much by bureaucracy as by medicine. In its thrust to science *DSM-IV* seeks to abolish mysteries and certainly to eschew speculative modes of thinking. The mysterious leap from mind to body that is the basis of psychosomatic disorders has disappeared from sight in favor of scientific pragmatism.

The reaction against the behaviorism of *DSM-III* and *IV* appears in a reiterated emphasis on the need for a holistic perception of the patient. The prime example of such a comprehensive vision is Engel's biopsychosocial model, discussed in chapter 1. Like Deutsch, Engel was a practicing internist who realized the limitations of exclusively somatic therapies and who therefore argued for a broader view that validated the psychological and the social aspects as directly relevant to the physical pathology, as the history of Mr. Glover's heart attacks shows. While Engel does not directly address the mystery of the leap from the mind to the body, his entire work devolves from acknowledgment of its potency.

If Engel has furnished the most fruitful clinical model, the most thoughtful cognitive work comes from Lipowski, a Polish-Canadian psychiatrist who specialized in liaison psychiatry, that is, the linkage of somatic medicine and psychiatry. The twenty-seven papers collected in his *Psychosomatic Medicine* (1985) date from 1967 to 1984. They address such topics as the history of the word "psychosomatic" (119–37), the epidemiological relationship between physical illness and psychiatric disorder (199–210), and the liaison of psychiatry with neurology and neurosurgery (365–72).

Lipowski's approach is the diametric opposite of that of *DSM*. He neither eschews the word "psychosomatic" nor does he seek to limit it to a restrictive definition. His working basis is remarkably open: "'*Psychosomatic*' is a term referring or related to the inseparability and interdependence of psychosocial and biologic (physiologic, somatic) aspects of humankind" (133). Lipowski considers the investigation of the psychosomatic as simultaneously a field, an approach, and a set of consulting activities. It is the unendingly puzzling and surprising nature of these disorders, their very elusiveness, that fascinates him. Lipowski's concept of the psychosomatic is far more intricate than that laid down in *DSM-IV*. Instead of pursuing narrow containment, Lipowski encourages an expansive stance by his refusal to segregate the psychosomatic and to perceive it only by default, as it were, in the appearance of complaints without an identifiable pathology. While he is bound, as a medical scientist, to try to fathom the mystery, he is also willing to grant the possibility of a residue not amenable to intellectual grasp.

Lipowski's major contribution lies in his ability to evolve a balanced and unified view of the psychosomatic without simplification and with due regard for its characteristic complexity. His fundamental tenet is the multicausality of disease; he envisages the possibility of a psychological component in any disease. In the emergence of psychosomatic complaints Lipowski attaches utmost importance to "intervening variables" (132) between the meaning imposed by individuals on information impinging on them and the somatic responses that follow. These intervening variables, expressed "through the mediation of neuroendocrine processes controlled by the brain," are determined by enduring personality dispositions and traits that reflect the patient's history, genetic endowment, and the experiences retained by memory. Decision conflicts, value conflicts, choices, threat, and loss are all to some degree innate to any disease state, and therefore apt to prompt psychic distress or psychological dysfunction. But it is in the patient's cognition and perception that the crucial psychological variables reside. Cutting through a tangle of what he dismisses as misconceptions, Lipowski proclaims his profound conviction that "a person is and responds as a unity" (5). The central function of psychosomatic medicine is thus "to study and to formulate explanatory hypotheses about the relationships between biological, psychological, and social phenomena as they pertain to persons" (5). The primary emphasis is constantly on the intervening variables and on the relationships between individuals as wholes in their interaction with the contexts in which they live and work, the adjustments and compromises they have continually to make, and how the pressures generated by the business of living, together with internal conflicts, affect their health.

In these transactions stress plays a leading part. It is defined "as *those social interactions and events as well as those psychological states that impose a burden on the organism by virtue of the emotions and the disturbances of body homeostasis that they elicit*" (114). The criteria for stress are multifaceted: it can originate within or outside the person; it must be experienced by the perceiving individual as threatening, although the process and the results of such an evaluation may be partly or totally beyond the person's awareness; the response must include one or more dysphoric affect as well as coping activities; the stress is felt, communicated, and described in psychological language. Stress can take many diverse forms: apart from injuries to the body, the frustration of drives, the loss or threat of loss of psychic objects (persons, ideals, bodily functions) or values, it may devolve from social changes that threaten a person's security. What matters most is the impact of the stress on the individual (what Lipowski calls "cognition and perception" [11]), especially any disproportion between the demands made and the power to deal with them without unreasonable or destructive costs. An overload of stress may induce "the giving-up-given-up complex" (41). The concomitants of stress (anxiety, depression, anger) have organismic effects that may prompt the onset of illness or foster its maintenance or exacerbation. Lipowski thus visualizes stress in a memorable image as "a series of linked and interacting loops" (17). The loops consist of affective arousal in response to the appraisal of a threat, which in turn influences cognitive processes in the direction of magnifying the threat with a resultant increase in affective arousal. The loop, or indeed the spiral, of stress is a vivid metaphor for the hidden mechanisms of the leap from mind to body.

All Lipowski's main ideas can be summarized under the adjective he most favors: "holistic." In pursuit of the holistic Lipowski advocates too the inclusion of environmental variables, "mind-body-environment interrela-tions," what he calls the "*ecological perspective*" (33). The gaze is thus expanded beyond the mind-body interrelation usually at the core of psy-chosomatic medicine. Environmental variables, Lipowski argues, play a part largely hitherto glossed over as sources of deprivation, temptation, loss, or danger that may trigger emotional responses and their physiologi-cal accompaniments.

The complex scenarios that emerge from the holistic, biopsychosocial method are "curvilinear"[18] rather than crudely linear in the manner of older attempts to establish direct psychogenic links between emotions and disturbances. "Curvilinear," in its suggestion of a winding path, invokes the notion of looping again. These innovative insights build on but also signif-icantly expand the earlier concept of the "stereoscopic picture" put for-ward by Dunbar. Like both Dunbar and Alexander, Lipowski is wholly committed to a monism devolving from the inseparability of mind and body. But unlike them, he draws less on Freudian concepts than on late twentieth-century thinking on ecological and environmental perspectives. He sees patients simultaneously as distinctive individuals and as enmeshed in the communities in which they live. This affirmation of the complicated nature of human existence shields Lipowski from the simplifying tendency to equate specific diseases (e.g., asthma, colitis) with certain personality traits. The canvas he presents in his *Psychosomatic Medicine* is considerably more subtle and multifaceted than previous work in the field. For that very reason, in confronting the mysterious connection between mind and body Lipowski desists from offering any solution to the puzzle. To him, in light of his firm belief in the essential cohesion of psyche and soma, it is to not so much a mysterious leap as an inevitable conjunction.

The inevitable nature of this conjunction is being probed by psychoneuro-biology and psychoneuroimmunology. Since the 1990s biomedical technol-ogy has been applied to mental health with the aim of exploring the biochemical mechanisms involved in conversion and other disorders as medical researchers have begun to examine the biochemical factors that impel that mysterious leap from mind to body. They hope to discover a cogent physical answer, as they succeeded in doing for epilepsy, which was long perceived as a primarily psychological malady, possibly related to the phases of the moon. Now it is classified as "a brain disorder" comprising both structural and biochemical aberrations.[19] For most disorders the picture remains less clear-cut, since emotional factors may coalesce with physically pathogenic agents in the causation of disease, with opinions oscillating at various times about the balance between the two. For example, peptic ulcer used to be regarded as a psychosomatic manifestation of stress. With the frequent finding of *H. pylori* bacteria in the stomachs of sufferers, it came to be attributed to an infection. Now this pathophysiology is being questioned again by a revival of the argument, made from a biopsychosocial point of view, that stress does play a significant role in the etiology of a number of cases that can be estimated as between 17 and 50 percent.[20]

Efforts to redefine the connection between psyche and soma utilizing scientifically convincing hypotheses have so far yielded only a few conclusive results. Stress hormones have been shown to have contradictory effects: on the one hand, in the short run they are useful in emergencies by diverting blood to the brain and muscles, at the expense of other tissues, to enable those in immediate danger to think and run more quickly. In the long run, on the other hand, the concomitant increased "stickiness" of the blood may eventually degrade the immune system, making tumors grow faster, causing brain damage and dementia as well as hardening of the arteries and spontaneous blood clots that lead to heart attacks and strokes.[21] Another connection between mental and physical states has been documented in levels of norephinephrine concentration in saliva and urine, an index of the arousal of the sympathetic nervous system, with higher levels corresponding to lower immune responses. The role of serotonin in body chemistry is also attracting much attention, but precisely how it works has not been fully fathomed. By and large the mediating mechanisms are far from completely understood as yet. The processes of the neuroendocrine system, in particular, have not been sufficiently explicated to map the pathways whereby the phase of feeling is attained. The study of neurotransmitters, and especially their interactions, amounts to a game of blind man's bluff. Nevertheless some psychiatrists, for instance, Steven Dubovsky in *Mind-Body Deceptions,* assert categorically that conversion disorders are produced through a physiological conduit via the brain. Mostly, however, the tone is more guarded and the wording quite tentative, often resorting to the term of uncertainty, "appear," or to phrasing such as "It is not unlikely that soon specific behaviors such as guilt, anger, and love will be explained by simple chemical processes."[22]

Endocrinology, as Freud foresaw, is indeed at the heels of analysis. In some areas, including obsessive-compulsive disorders and endogenous depression, innate biochemical triggers are being postulated, since these illnesses respond to corrective chemical input. But no firm evidence of this kind exists to account for psychosomatic disorders. They still represent a rather mysterious leap from mind to body.

CHAPTER FOUR

Literary Patients

I know that's a secret for it's whispered everywhere.
　　　　　　　　　　　　　—Congreve, *Love for Love*

"The psychiarist who takes it upon himself to attempt a character study of an individual whom he has never met is engaged upon a project which is full of risk."[1] With these words the eminent British psychiatrist Anthony Storr expresses his reservations at the opening of his study, "Churchill's Black Dog, Kafka's Mice, and Oher Phenomena of the Human Mind." He goes on to elaborate on the difficulty of assessing a person (Churchill) whom he never actually met: "In the exercise of his profession, the psychiatrist has an unrivaled opportunity for the appraisal of character, and may justly claim that he knows more persons deeply and intimately than most of his fellows. But, when considering someone who has died, he is deprived of those special insights which can only be attained in the consulting room, and is, like the historian, obliged to rely upon what written evidence happens to be available" (3).

Storr's astute speculations about Churchill have an illustrious precedent in Freud's "Psychoanalytische Bemerkungen über einen autobiographisch beschriebenen Fall von Paranoia (Dementia Paranoides)" (1911; "Psychoanalytic Notes upon an Autobiographical Account of a Case of Paranoia [Dementia Paranoides]). Like Storr with Churchill, Freud never met the lawyer, Daniel Schreber, who published his *Denkwürdigkeiten eines Nervenkranken* (Memoirs of a Neurotic) in 1903. Freud is not even sure whether Schreber was still alive in 1911; he appears to have made no attempt to follow up personally on Schreber, basing his analysis exclusively on the written evidence Schreber had left behind. Yet Freud evidently feels a certain need to justify his psychoanalysis of this patient he had never seen, just as Storr does in regard to Churchill. He points out that a physician like himself who is not attached to a public institution does not have long-term

53

access to cases of paranoia. But he believes it is "nicht . . . unstatthaft"[2] (not inadmissible) to practice an analytic interpretation on Schreber because he had written and published his own case history.[3] The English translation of "nicht . . . unstatthaft" as "legitimate" (104) is far more positive than Freud's formulation, a double negative that projects a certain hesitancy.

Although both Freud and Storr reflect on the risks innate to probing a patient who cannot be and has not been present in the customary face-to-face situation in the consulting room, both decide nonetheless to go ahead, substituting written evidence for the direct encounter. Storr, who also draws on testimony from Churchill's family and friends, emphasizes that "what I have to say must be regarded as tentative" (4). He illustrates "the possibilities of error" by referring to the "disastrous study of Woodrow Wilson" (4) by Freud and William Bullitt.

These caveats must arouse apprehensions in the literary critic who embarks on a psychiatric reading of a figure in a novel or a play. Storr is concerned about dealing with a person who has died and Freud with one who has disappeared, whereas the literary critic examines a character who has never actually lived. However, psychological studies of characters in literature are already well established as an effective way of analyzing the protagonists' motivations as well as the dynamics among the figures.[4] What is more, psychological interactions including decision conflicts, family strife, obsessive-compulsive tendencies, and depressive feelings are part of everyone's life and may escalate almost imperceptibly from a normal to a debilitating level.[5] Still, the critic who sets out to examine psychosomatic disorders in literary works must weigh the risks against the rewards of considering literary figures as patients.

The risks are more readily apparent than the rewards. The very fictitiousness of the characters seems a primary stumbling block. Unlike Churchill and Schreber, literary patients have never existed and have left no written evidence of their own on which to base an interpretation. The only real quality that a fictional character can authentically be said to possess is an essentially literary one, such as appearing in chapter 3. When Dickens describes Mrs. Gamp as being fat, it is a property that he has invented and ascribed to her. Our belief in her fatness depends on one of the fundamental conventions of reading. Coleridge's phrase, "a willing suspension of disbelief for the moment"[6] is frequently cited, although in regard to realistic works it is more pertinent to speak of readers' willingness to pretend belief for the moment.[7] If we are able to pretend to believe in characters' existence at all (as we clearly do for the span of our reading and even

beyond), that belief will also encompass—apart from the qualities attributed to them, such as fatness—various other aspects of their lives: their
loves, their desires, their fears, their marriages, their illnesses, and their
deaths. The characters' feelings of happiness or distress thus attain a temporary and provisional realness through our constructive acts of reading.

To acknowledge the essential fictitiousness of literary characters does
not entail a radical discontinuity between the worlds outside and within the
fiction. In realist fiction, founded as it is on observation of prevailing mores
and lifestyles, the adjacent realms run parallel. Close observation, careful
documentation, and frequently personal familiarity with the arena of the
action on the writer's part were the pillars of the realists' and naturalists'
writings. Although characters and their problems were not usually modeled directly on identifiable individuals, they are chosen as typifying a
common fate under the circumstances of that particular time and place.[8]

Social observation also provided images of illness. It is striking, however, that much illness in fiction is rather indefinite. What, for instance, ails
Squire Hamley's wife in Elizabeth Gaskell's *Wives and Daughters* (1866)? Mr.
Gibson, the family doctor, is in constant attendance on her through years
of invalidism, and eventually she dies without any indication of the nature
of her chronic affliction. Similarly, we can only guess at the malady of
another literary patient in Oliver Wendell Holmes's *Elsie Venner* (1861). Perhaps she suffers from tuberculosis, a great scourge at that time, especially
among young women, but Holmes never alludes to coughing, or palor, or
emaciation. Even more puzzling is the spate of brain fevers. Apart from
those already mentioned in chapter 2, this phenomenon occurs in two of
Conan Doyle's stories, "Naval Treaty" (1892) and "Copper Beeches"
(1892). Though himself a physician, Conan Doyle unhesitatingly accepts
this nebulous malady. One way to account for the absence of specificity in
the illnesses of many nineteenth-century literary patients is by reference to
the relative lack of precise information prior to the development of
modern understandings of disease and modern diagnostic methods. From
a literary perspective, a sudden illness such as brain fever may be a plot
device. As Audrey Peterson suggests, in Elizabeth Gaskell's *Ruth* (1853),
"Mr. Bellingham develops brain fever at a point in the novel when his illicit
affair with Ruth needs to be terminated."[9] So it is a convenient means of
disposing of a character who has become superfluous. In *Madame Bovary*
Emma's attack serves to show her husband's great tenderness toward her.
In Conan Doyle's "Naval Treaty," the nine weeks Percy Phelps lies unconscious corresponds to the time a secret government document remains
missing and so aggravates the seriousness of the case.

Partly perhaps because of the impossibility of more exact diagnosis,
writers relied on the holistic assumptions of the period, not only recording

the course of illnesses but also making connections between mind and body. In *The Bride of Lammermoor* (1819) Scott coins the graphic phrase "a fever upon the spirit"[10] to denote Lucy Ashton's frenzied state in the novel's Gothic culminating scene. Her physical disarray ("her head gear dishevelled—her night-clothes torn and dabbed with blood—her eyes glazed, and her features convulsed" [260]) is presented as the visible manifestation of her emotional turbulence as she feels "beset on all hands, and in a manner reduced to despair" (238). The popular and vague nineteenth-century notion of "fever," including so-called brain fever, is here directly linked to Lucy's mental extremity, delineating an integral association between psyche and soma. The fact that Lucy exists only in Scott's novel—and consequently in our imagination—does not detract from the vividness of the representation that disposes readers to believe in it.

The conjunction of physical and psychological disorders is portrayed with equal credibility in a number of nineteenth-century fictions as the product of perspicacious social observation. While the protagonists in such novels as Charlotte Brontë's *Shirley* and Balzac's *Le Cousin Pons* (discussed in chapter 2) are, of course, fictitious, their predicaments replicate archetypal human dilemmas, and so they partake of a wider truthfulness that extends beyond the limits of the fiction. This holds too for the patterns of their illnesses, which conform to a large degree to the findings of modern medicine.[11] The terminology has changed; Scott's "fever upon the spirit" now sounds archaically fanciful, and the word "nervous" has become so vague as to forfeit much of its force. But the presence of psychological components is quite pronounced. And the characters' anxieties, their despondencies, their griefs, voiced and unvoiced, like their loves and hopes, though obviously fictitious, are also recognizable as universal human experiences.

The cardinal problem or risk in constructing illnesses in fictional characters stems not so much from their fictitiousness as from the literary configuration in which readers meet them. By literary configuration I mean above all the mediation of the patient by the narrator or dramatist. Even if the animator of the fiction remains hidden, refraining from direct comment or intervention, an intermediary is nevertheless inevitably inserted between character and reader. In this respect the literary situation departs most markedly from that in clinical practice, where the physician sees (in the widest sense) the patient, and also from that of Storr with Churchill and Freud with Schreber, since both could draw on their respective subjects' own writings. The literary disposition precludes such direct access to the figure; readers' knowledge is circumscribed, determined by what narrator or dramatist wishes us to know. The possibilities of manipulation must therefore always be kept in mind, for the writer may be sympathetic, or ironic, or ambivalent toward the protagonist he or she is portraying. The issue of the degree of reliability or unreliability of the narrating voice is particularly acute in first-person narration, where the speaker may engage in deception or self-deception. Paradoxically, however, this is the point where the literary configuration approximates most closely to that in clinical practice, for the patient may also consciously or unconsciously resort to obfuscation, withholding or distorting crucial information.

To some degree all patients will, without deliberate intent, engage in such misrepresentation. For instance, depressives will overstate the difficulties facing them in a pessimistically negative assessment of their situation. Conversely, manics will minimize those same difficulties in optimistic overconfidence. The psychiatrist's task is to correct those exaggerations by means of a "reality check." Seated face to face with the patient, and trained in observation, the psychiatrist will read the patient's condition from his or her voice, body language, and expression that will—as much as the words uttered—reveal mutedness, despondency, excitement, or agitation.

Literary patients, by contrast, are not present face to face; they can be perceived only through the intermedium of the printed word. But texts emit signals that correspond to the patient's tone of voice, expression, and so on. They, too, project a distinctive tone, be it of skepticism or tenderness, and they comprise certain strategies that alert readers to read between the lines in the same way as psychiatrists do. Such literary tactics as irony, satire, parody, caricature, internal contradictions, and gaps indicate the precariousness of what is being said. Like the experienced psychiatrist, the competent reader will spot these strategies and construct the words in keeping with the covert instructions encoded in the verbal fabric. Nevertheless, the literary patient's greater remoteness from the reader than the actual patient's opposite the psychiatrist is an added complication. The interposition of the writer between character and reader results in a triangulated relationship.

The two most common configurations that arouse doubts are either a distancing from the literary patient or its inverse, an excessive closeness. Distancing fosters suspense and bewilderment. For example, in Emily Brontë's *Wuthering Heights* (1847), the story of Catherine Linton is recounted to Mr. Lockwood by Nelly Dean, the housekeeper. As a newcomer to the area, Mr. Lockwood functions as a surrogate listener, with whom readers identify in their curiosity to learn what goes on in the remote, uncanny house. The estranging physical environment is evoked through the outsider's unsettling perceptions even before Nelly's narration. Mr. Lockwood's initial encounter with Wuthering Heights prepares readers for the bizarre happenings at the house. The novel's very title, immediately suggests an ominous aura: "'Wuthering' being a significant provincial adjective, descriptive of the atmospheric tumult to which its station is exposed in stormy weather."[12] Taking shelter from a sudden snowstorm, Mr. Lockwood finds the place eerie and its inhabitants moody and unfriendly. In recalling the experience the next day, he shudders at the thought of "that bleak hilltop," the "heath and mud," "misty and cold" (14), and even on his obligatory thank-you call, "the dismal spiritual atmosphere overcame, and more than neutralized, the glowing physical comforts round me" (20).

So Nelly Dean's narrative is embedded in a setting already rife with suspicion and malaise. Although Nelly was an eyewitness to the events she reports, the trustworthiness of her testimony must be questioned, since she is a dismissed servant who clearly harbors strong likes and dislikes. Her intermediacy as the storyteller opens up a space of contingency that readers, with Mr. Lockwood, can fill only with conjecture. The mysteriousness of Catherine's collapse and death is intensified by the paucity of assured evidence. The murkiness, both physical and psychological, in which the narrative is enveloped, is a primary source of its fascination. That penumbra is a direct product of its narrative disposition; the dual frame of Mr. Lockwood and Nelly Dean keeps the central characters and happenings at a remove from readers. Yet these very narrational devices that make *Wuthering Heights* so endlessly intriguing also engender a considerable risk for a reading of Catherine's illness, which always remains beyond our ken. Thus this Gothic tale casts us as perplexed spectators of a drama we may experience with a shudder but can never wholly understand.

A similar distancing is pushed to extremes in Bram Stoker's *Dracula* (1897). The intricacy of its series of frames has provoked the criticism that it is an "over-complicated narrative,"[13] yet precisely those complications in the telling serve the purpose of compounding the perplexities of deciphering Jonathan's weird encounters and thereby heighten the horror. News of his sudden, violent illness comes to his fiancée, Mina Murray, in a letter from Sister Agatha that is interpolated into Mina's journal. This letter is only one of several very disparate documents incorporated into the journal: a cutting from the *Daily Telegraph* of 8 August about a storm and a shipwreck; excerpts from the "Log of the 'Demeter,'" translated from Russian, and letters exchanged between lawyers in London and Whitby about shipments. The status of these documents and their inclusion in Mina's journal is puzzling until the mosaic pieces of the plot fall into place much later in the narrative. Sister Agatha's letter from the hospital of St. Joseph and St. Mary, Budapest, dated 12 August and directed to Miss Wilhelmina Murray about her fiancé's brain fever is more immediately grounded. Yet even though there is no intrinsic reason to doubt Sister Agatha's declarative testimony, its insertion into a curious assortment of cryptic reports taints its credibility. As in *Wuthering Heights,* readers' narrational remove from the character's illness increases the riskiness of constructing it.

At the opposite extreme to these mediated accounts are the subjective versions offered by the patients themselves. Percy Phelps in Conan Doyle's "The Adventure of the Naval Treaty" tells his own story to Dr. Watson in the first person: "I had a fit in the station, and before we reached home I was practically a raving maniac. . . . Here I have lain, Mr. Holmes, for over nine weeks, unconscious and raving with brain fever. . . . Slowly my reason has cleared, but it is only in the last three days that my memory has quite returned."[14] Phelps's loss of consciousness and of memory obviously precludes any particularized description of his attack. Jeanne's situation in Maupassant's *Une Vie* (1883; *A Woman's Life*) is similar, although the narrative is cast in indirect discourse focalized from her point of view. After collapsing in the snow and being rescued by members of her household, she recalls only "un cauchemar" (a nightmare) and is not sure whether it was a nightmare in the normal sense.[15] She remembers the sensation of mice running all over her and "une douleur horrible" (113; a horrible pain). As she recovers, she finds that many things escape her because of gaps in her memory. Likewise for readers, Jeanne's illness is full of gaps. So, too great a closeness to the protagonist has ultimately the same effect as too great a distance: the illness remains shadowy, a will-o'-the-wisp presence to be glimpsed but not amenable to more direct scrutiny.

The uncertainty intrinsic to enframed or first-person narratives is a factor, to a lesser extent, in all literary texts because they are aesthetic artifacts fashioned by an author. The information about the characters available to readers is determined by the author's choices. Unlike the physician in the consulting room, readers cannot further probe possibly important areas that remain veiled within the fiction. In George Eliot's *Middlemarch* (1872), for instance, we are told that Lydgate was orphaned in adolescence when his father died. How old was he when his mother died? What is the gender of his two siblings? Did he have a good or a bad relationship to his guardian's wife? Answers to these questions might help us to account for Lydgate's repeatedly poor judgments of women, a personal failing in such glaring contrast to his fine professional judgment. Perhaps a lack of contact with women during his formative years deprived him of the experience to make wiser decisions in adulthood. We can do no more than speculate because Eliot has not addressed these matters. Readers are thus at the mercy of the author's selectivity, a prerogative that circumscribes our knowledge. While some works encourage reading *between* the lines by suggesting the unreliability of the narrating voice, reading *beyond* the lines amounts to mere invention on the reader's part, a transgression of the boundaries that we as readers have to accept.

The elusiveness of the reading process parallels the elusiveness of psychosomatic disorders. Like the physician in pursuit of a diagnosis, the reader is committed to a task of detection in sifting the clues to the most appropriate construction of the text. The problem of uncertainty in diagnosing a psychosomatic disorder coincides with the analogous difficulty of attaining an assured reading of a text. Multiple possibilities and perspectives abound in both situations, so that definitive truth is hard to ascertain. The succession of contradictory (and self-contradictory) first-person narrators in Brian O'Doherty's *Strange Case of Mademoiselle P.,* the divergent versions of the Gellburgs' marriage in Arthur Miller's *Broken Glass,* the ambiguity of the images of Thomas in Thomas Mann's *Buddenbrooks:* these are examples of the literary tactics of uncertainty that correspond to the uncertainties characteristic of psychosomatic disorders.

However, the divergence of the medium between medicine and literature creates another dimension of risk in the analysis of an unseen, that is, a literary patient. In medicine, Barbour asserts, "body language is eloquent, and forces the issue";[16] the body becomes language, a means of expressing distress in conversion disorders. Freud's patient with the facial neuralgia had translated the pain of a slap in the face inflicted on her into a recurrent physical sensation of pain in that spot. The mysterious leap, the conversion from psyche to soma is here quite transparent. But a further conversion has to take place in the literary work: into language. Storr with Churchill, largely, and Freud with Schreber, entirely, rely on their subjects' own words. In fiction and drama what we have are the author's words, attributed to the protagonists. So in the literary portrayal of conversion disorders, a dual translation occurs: from the fictional character's mind into his/her body and also into the linguistic medium of the text. As for Storr and Freud, the foundational material is a verbal sequence that delineates and represents a human being. This verbalization inevitably results in simultaneous closeness and distancing. Either way there are risks.

Why, then, in the face of these acknowledged risks engage in studies of psychosomatic disorders in literary patients? Because the arguments in favor of such an enterprise are strong: despite undeniable drawbacks, literary portrayals also have important features conducive to a deeper insight into psychosomatic disorders, particularly into their etiology.

Foremost among these is the suitability of literary works for the application of the biopsychosocial model. This model places major emphasis on what Lipowski calls the "intervening variables."[17] These comprise social situations and life events as well as personality traits, psychological states, behaviors, and subjective perceptions, all of which may prove to contribute to a wide range of anomalies in health. The crux of psychosomatic disorders lies in the "interactional aspects of man's functioning," "mind-body-environment relations."[18]

These are the very areas in which literary works can excel. The strength of literary portrayals lies in their capacity for amplitude in space, time, and motivation. In their potential for social and temporal expansiveness, they can show the processes whereby psychosomatic disorders unfold in the context of the interactions and conflicts that shape a person's responses, and they can do so over the lengthy time span of the many years that may precede the eventual emergence of the disturbance. By its nature literature is able to offer case histories that reach back to the origins of the disorder rather than just case studies of the current symptoms. More than medical science, literature can track "the mysterious leap" by depicting the griefs and stresses, the chain of experiences that prompt the leap. It is well to recall here that Barbour at the Stanford Diagnostic Clinic had to resort to words, to "just talk"[19] after a host of medical tests and procedures had failed to produce a viable diagnosis, let alone an understanding of his patients' complaints. The verbal medium, as Freud found out in "the talking cure," is that most suited to what Josef Breuer's patient, Anna O dubbed "chimney sweeping," the dredging up of the psychological problems known to underlie psychosomatic disorders.

Among Lipowski's "intervening variables," the one more easily accessible to the writer than to the clinician is the patient's social context. Whereas physicians see patients in the neutral zone of the consulting room, generally alone, and only occasionally with a family member or members, writers delight in the liberty of filling out a rich picture of their protagonists' environment: the places where they live, the furnishings of their houses, their prized possessions, their occupations, their financial standing, their status in the community, their leisure activities, their reading preferences, and so on. Apart from these concrete details, the moral aspects of the characters' milieu, too, form a vital facet of this picture: the ethos of their time and place, the behavioral expectations held before them as, for instance, women, or younger sons, or ministers of religion, the life paths they are supposed to follow in accordance with their station on the social ladder. Such words as "expectations" and "supposed to follow" already suggest the pressures that may be exerted by their social position. When societal pressures contravene individual desires, the scene is set for conflicts, both intrapersonal and interpersonal. For the individual may suppress his or her wishes—and frequently it is a woman who does so—in order to conform to the approved pattern, or even if she inwardly rebels against it, may opt for the ease of a surface conformity that masks the rebellion. Whatever the choice, and whether it is conscious or unconscious, distress will surely ensue in the long run, if not at once.

Such social and environmental variables, Lipowski argues, can trigger a spectrum of feelings according to personality and situation.[20] They may be experienced as sources of deprivation or temptation, loss or danger, and so elicit a variety of emotional responses and their physiological concomitants. Psychic distress and physiological dysfunction may emanate from decision conflicts, value conflicts, conflicts about the approach/avoidance alternative, a discrepancy between hopes and gratification, all of which may mobilize ego defenses that may be turned outward or inward. Turned outward, the aggression is likely further to intensify the strife between the individual and his/her environment to an explosive climax. On the other hand, inhibitions to the expression of unavowed or disavowed feelings are liable to trigger conversion from mind to body as an oblique outlet for the repressed hurt.

Since they are a primary element in the social environment, relationships with other human beings are a decisive factor. Wittingly or unwittingly, others may be the cause of tensions and stress. Alexander affirms the synthesis in the psychosomatic approach between "the individual's relation to his social environment" and "internal physiological processes."[21] Even more categorically Arthur Kleinman states that "the family is often a major player in the illness drama."[22] His use of the literary term "drama" makes a striking connection between medicine and literature.

Disruptions of established relationships through death, or divorce, or suspicion of one partner's having an affair, or a move to another locale, or changes in the work environment, or children growing up and claiming independence may be antecedents to illness. Such changes may on the surface appear pleasant (e.g., a promotion at work), or perfectly normal (e.g., adolescents going away to college), yet turn out to be upsetting by imposing an additional burden of responsibility or leaving an "empty nest" that may manifest in anxiety and depression respectively. Marital, occupational, and social problems are found in association with anxiety, depression, phobias, and substance abuse in at least 50 percent of conversion disorders.[23] Dependency, voluntary or instilled, is another frequent source of difficulties. In the biopsychosocial model, unsuccessful coping, incapacities, and maladaptive behaviors in the social context play a role as important as the intrapsychic conflicts that were the center of interest for Alexander and his fellow psychoanalysts. In relationships and behaviors, writers have a distinct advantage over physicians. Clinicians are obliged skillfully and at times laboriously to elicit from patients information about the tensions in their environment and relationships. Patients may be either reluctant to disclose details or unaware of the destructive impact of their own habitual behavior or of that of those in their family and surroundings. Here, as I have argued, the clinician resembles the reader of a literary work in having to read between the lines so as to construct the realities of the patient's life. No such barriers impede writers. They know whatever they wish about their characters and let be known as much as they choose. The advantages of the literary configuration come to the fore here. Even when narrators pretend not to be omniscient, the very gaps and omissions in their accounts may be indirectly telling in prompting readers to reconsider the overt version. Some writers, in order to know their own protagonists more thoroughly, have sketched in preparatory notebooks complete life histories that go well beyond the information necessary to the plot. Emile Zola, for example, established each figure's *état civil* (social state) and drew up a family tree of all the major members of the two branches in his *Rougon-Macquart* cycle (1871–93) to document their heredity and interconnections as well as their occupations, physical features, and personality traits. In her *Quarry for "Middlemarch"* George Eliot went so far as to delineate characters who never appear in the novel so as to command a total overview of the lives of her protagonists.

From the vantage point of this unlimited stock of information about their protagonists, writers can represent relationships with as much density and vividness as environment: family strife in *The Strange Case of Mademoiselle P.*, generational discord and sibling rivalries in *Buddenbrooks*, marital unhappiness in *Broken Glass*, disappointed love in *Thérèse Raquin*, betrayals in *The Scarlet Letter*. Above all, literary works, instead of only telling about these happenings, actually *show* how they occur and how they affect the protagonists' feelings about themselves and those involved with them. Such enactment before readers' eyes produces a far livelier image than mere recital, and invites readers' participation as if they themselves were voyeuristic spectators of the scenes being played out before them. This strategy of showing enables readers to watch, as it were, the circumstances leading up to the psychosomatic disorder.

These circumstances can more easily be traced in literary works than in clinical practice because literature often covers an extensive time span in a character's life and so can follow the unfolding of an emotional disorder. *Buddenbrooks*, for instance, spans the forty years between 1835 and 1875; the last section of *Mademoiselle P.* is dated thirty-seven years after the first four; *The Scarlet Letter*, judging by Pearl's growing up, extends over ten years or more. Even when the focus is on the moment of crisis, a retrospect on the earlier events that culminate in the crisis is almost always opened up. *Broken Glass* uncovers recollections of over twenty years on the Gellburgs' marriage; similarly, *Regeneration* reconstructs the events and experiences that have led up to and contributed causally to the current crisis. In all these instances, the retrospect provides the key to the psychological distress, although it may require interpretation on the part of readers who are made to act as sleuths. Indeed, nearly all literary portrayals of psychosomatic disorders take the form of detective stories, with the illness as the mystery to be unraveled. For it is in the past, as psychoanalysis insists, that the source of the disorder lies and there that it has to be ferreted out. Literary works flesh out the possibilities of the biopsychosocial model through their extensive time span which allows the tracing of the gradual growth of conflicted relationships.

The literary work can also map in the vicissitudes of the plot the correlation between the time and place of the onset of the physical symptoms, their exacerbation, remissions, and relapses to external (social) and internal (psychological) conditions. Psychiatrists are in agreement on this correlation. Alexander recommends special attention to the chronological sequence, reasoning that the study of "precursory, often transitory symptoms in earlier age periods shows that they develop during times of emotional stress and disappear with the relief of the emotional tension, only to recur whenever new conflict situations arise under the vicissitudes of life."[24] *DSM-IV*, too underscores that observation of "a close temporal relationship between a conflict or stressor and the initiation or exacerbation of a symptom may be helpful in this determination [the diagnosis of a conversion disorder], especially if the person has developed conversion symptoms under similar circumstances in the past" (453–54). The dynamics, spatial, social, and temporal pivotal to the biopsychosocial model, parallel the development of plot in literary works and so make them a particularly rewarding vehicle for the analysis of psychosomatic disorders.

What is more, the subjective element that Lipowski calls "cognition and perception"[25] is wide open to understanding in literary works because of their capacity to switch the point of view. In his awareness of individual as well as environmental variables Lipowski notes that the source of distress differs from one person to another. The meanings of certain events and reactions to them are shaped by enduring personality traits which reflect the person's history, genetic endowment, and experiences retained by memory. All these factors in combination codetermine how life situations and changes are likely to be appraised, and what emotions they will activate. These emotions, together with the associated memories, can be directly revealed in the literary practice of entering into the characters' minds, in such techniques as indirect discourse or stream of consciousness. So the etiology of the psychosomatic disorder can be illuminated from within, from the sufferer's perspective, in contrast to the physician's view presented in the medical textbooks. The sufferer's repressions and denials, the efforts to avoid or escape the issue can be implied too. This is another major gain to be reaped from the study of psychosomatic disorders in literature.

All in all, the application of the biopsychosocial model to literature illustrates the innate metaphoricity of its three associated strands. The overt physical symptom, puzzling to physicians because of the absence of an ascertainable pathology, functions as the flag to signal distress. The symptom is a cipher, a veiled externalization of inner pain. The social dimension acts as a trigger, precipitating a crisis in the wake of the individual's interactions with his or her environment. The circumstances that bring matters to a head may be either the cumulative pressure of a long-term situation or a sudden incident, or, frequently, a combination of the two when a particular episode escalates a previously tolerated discontent to an intolerable pitch. This social transaction is a circular process, a spiral of stress loops that double back on themselves until the loop winds up as an intractable knot. The ulterior conflict may have simmered for a considerable time, more or less endured—and/or ignored—by those involved, as in a marital maladjustment, or a sibling rivalry, or a generational discord, until abruptly, sometimes at an apparently slight provocation, it is transformed from a chronic tension into an acute conversion disorder. So, while the symptom is the external manifestation, the core of the disorder is an internal, displaced distress. Repressed, unavowed, effaced from the sufferer's consciousness, the psychological hurt is a secret hidden from the self as well as from others, that surfaces solely in its converted physical form.

The secret at the core of psychosomatic disorders is contained in the presenting complaint. "To contain" denotes at once to hold out and to hold back. The ostensible symptom both indicates and screens the secret, which has to be mined and deciphered. The closest analogy is the interpretation of dreams. For "psychosomatic symptoms always carry a message. All of them serve the same purpose: escape from a difficult, embarrassing, or painful situation."[26] Or, as Deutsch puts it, "[T]he conversion symptom acts as a protective mechanism, the action of which is the equivalent to the amount of anxiety to be prevented."[27] Barbour, too, realizes that the questions the physician must ask are: "What are the patient's needs? What is the inner meaning of the message? What situation forces the problem to take this form?"[28] The symptoms allow a partial expression in disguise of feelings such as aggression, or instinctive impulses, for instance of a sexual nature, that the patient regards as socially prohibited.[29]

The concept of the conversion symptom as a symbolic pointer to a secret has a lengthy history. Freud envisaged bodily symptoms as directly symbolic of the original conflict; the clearest example is the patient who converted a slap in the face into recurrent, recalcitrant attacks of facial neuralgia. In support of the symbolizing hypothesis Freud also observed that the site of the conversion disorder frequently coincided with that of a previous physical injury or illness; Elisabeth von R . . . in *Studies on Hysteria* experiences psychosomatic pain in her legs where she had had a rheumatic episode. Among Freud's followers, Alexander is most emphatic in his endorsement of this view: "A conversion symptom is a *symbolic* expression of an emotionally charged psychological content."[30] The editors (Harold Kaplan, Benjamin Sadock, and Jack Grebb) of the *Synopsis of Psychiatry*, too, underscore the symbolic value of the symptom as a representation of an unconscious pyschological conflict (622). The primary gain to patients is to keep internal conflicts beyond their awareness by projecting outward, almost as an instinctive self-protection.[31]

The central role of the secret in the formation of neuroses was posited before Freud by another Viennese physician, Moritz Benedikt (1835–1920). In a series of publications between 1864 and 1895 Benedikt "showed that the cause of many cases of hysteria and other neuroses resides in a painful secret, mostly pertaining to sexual life, and that many patients can be cured by the confession of their pathogenic secrets and by the working out of the related problems."[32] But even before Benedikt, the therapeutic, cathartic effects of speaking out a disturbing secret had been institutionalized in the Protestant practice of *Seelensorge* (care of the soul) which arose after reformers had abolished compulsory confession. Certain Protestant ministers were considered to be endowed with a spiritual gift that enabled them to obtain confession of a troubling secret from distressed souls and so to help them out of their difficulty.[33] However, in such religious confession, the subject must beforehand be aware of his or her own secret. By contrast, in a conversion disorder the secret is precisely what the sufferer represses, banishing it from consciousness and supplanting it into the body. Dora, Freud notes at one stage in her analysis, "deckt wiederum ein ganzes Stück ihrer eigenen geheimen Geschichte" ("concealed a whole section of her secret history").[34] She is at pains "das Geheimnis nicht [zu] verraten" ("not to betray her secret").[35] That repressed secret has been deemed to act "like a psychic poison."[36]

The psychological as well as the moral implications of secrets are the subject of Sissela Bok's *Secrets: On the Ethics of Concealment and Revelation*. Although she concentrates primarily on the ethical and interpersonal aspects, she also opens up large vistas onto thorny intrapersonal issues. Taking as her starting point the myth of Pandora's box, she comments that "the question whether to leave evil secrets alone or try to defeat them by draining them of their destructive power recurs in many therapeutic and investigative practices" (4). She recognizes the secret as "set apart in the mind of its keeper as requiring concealment" (5). Often the purpose of such concealment is social, to protect others from discomfiting information. But it may also serve to protect the self: "[S]elf-deception may be our only shield against knowledge that would otherwise cripple us. . . . In deceiving ourselves . . . we keep secret from ourselves the truth we cannot face" (60). Significantly, Bok uses the word "cripple," for that is precisely what a psychosomatic disorder may do even as it functions as a shield against, or a distracting conversion of, knowledge that cannot be faced.

So silence is, as Bok puts it, "the first defense of secrets" (7). This is conveyed in the Greek word *arretos*, which originally meant just the unspoken but later also referred to "the unspeakable, the ineffable, the prohibited, sometimes also the abominable and shameful" (7). Since concealment is the defining trait of secrecy, it results in the separation between insider and outsider: "[T]o think something secret," Bok argues, "is already to envisage potential conflict between what insiders conceal and outsiders want to inspect or lay bare" (6). But Bok does not envisage the possibility that insiders and outsiders may be one and the same person, simultaneously wanting to hide and to expose. If the emotional charge of the pathogenic secret, turned outward, may find expression in anger, aggression against others, destructiveness, turned inward against the self, it may be converted into a bodily pain that is at once self-destructive and self-defensive. Flight from the secret into illness is in effect a means of acknowledging the presence of a problem by displacing it into a culturally more acceptable area.

The paradox intrinsic to the tricky balance between concealment and revelation, particularly in relation to our selves, is a problem to Bok. She designates as "tantalizing" the hints "at powers intending to keep us in the dark. A hidden intention may be at play—most paradoxical of all when it is taken to be our own intention to forget and to keep knowledge at arm's length" (10). Repeatedly she returns to "the paradox of both knowing and not knowing the same thing at the same time" (63), seeing it as a mode of self-deception in which "a split self or even several selves are at work . . . to guard against anxiety-producing knowledge" (63). Bok remains troubled by this paradox: "[H]ow can one be both insider and outsider thus, keeping secrets from oneself, even lying to oneself? How can one simultaneously know and ignore the same thing?" (61).

One response to this paradox—one that Bok does not mention—is in somatization. By converting the secret from psychological into physical distress, we satisfy the need that Bok perceives "to hide and to share" (xvi). The psychosomatic disorder represents a means of fulfilling that dual and contradictory urge simultaneously to know and not to know, indeed to *display* and to *conceal*.

This tension between knowing and not knowing, concealment and revelation finds a culturally acceptable mode of expression in psychosomatic disorders. At the conscious level, patients literally do not know their distress; unconsciously, they reveal in their bodily symptoms what they need to conceal from themselves. The secret thus corresponds to the wish or the fear at the heart of the dream as the latent propellant to the conversion process. Speaking through the body is a means to reconcile concealment and revelation, for the distress is unmistakably put forth while the secret itself stays safely hidden.

The excavation of such pathogenic secrets is one of the major aims of the "talking cure" and its various precursors.[37] They rest on the recognition of the therapeutic value of speaking out and thereby confronting and ultimately working through unpalatable truths. By means of the strategy of free association, psychoanalysis induces patients to utter whatever is passing through their minds and so to provide clues about anguish relegated to the unconscious. The astutely listening analyst's task is to pick up these involuntarily yielded clues, to trace them back to their original source, and to make the analysand aware of the initiating trauma. In this sense psychoanalysis and its successor, psychotherapy, amounts to an attempted exorcism of the troubling but unavowed distress.

But psychotherapeutic care is not universally available—or invariably successful. Bok argues that undiscovered secrets, the product of lies (as much to ourselves as to others) "build up" (xv). Or perhaps it would be more appropriate to say that they burrow down, sapping and undermining the individuals who guard them. In order to avoid total collapse, and at the same time to solicit help, they replace verbalization by speaking through the body, exhibiting a psychosomatic disorder as an overt idiom of distress that functions as a substitute—and cover—for the buried secret.

Literary patients afford insight into the mechanisms of hide-and-seek instrumental in the formation of psychosomatic disorders. They are portrayed in their social environment as members of distinctive families and communities that often are a central factor in the distressing situations with which they are increasingly unable to deal. The history of their difficulties emerges either in a plot that spans many years, as in *The Scarlet Letter* and *Buddenbrooks,* or as a retrospective uncovering of mounting tensions in the past prior to the outbreak of the illness, as in *Broken Glass, The Strange Case of Mademoiselle P.,* and *Regeneration.* Common to all the literary patients, whatever their actual symptoms—paralysis, blindness, multiple neurological symptoms, and so forth—is their avoidance of a pain that has become intolerable. A cardinal motif is therefore that of silence as an indicator of the repression of secrets harbored in a blend of social and self-deception.

These themes of societal pressures, avoidance, guilt of various kinds, silence and secrecy crop up in a spectrum of diverse works with a wide temporal range. The recurrence of similar elements under different guises in very heterogeneous works bears out the view of psychosomatic disorders catalogued in medical textbooks. At the same time, and more important, it offers a complementary humanistic understanding of the crises that are precipitated into such disorders. The secrets of the literary patients are "whispered everywhere" throughout the texts.

PART II

Metaphors of Distress

CHAPTER FIVE

"A Strange Sympathy
betwixt Soul and Body"

Nathaniel Hawthorne, *The Scarlet Letter* (1850)

> This is his first punishment, that by the verdict of his
> own heart no guilty man is acquitted.
>
> —Juvenal, *Satires*

The phrase "a strange sympathy betwixt soul and body," which so aptly characterizes the essence of psychosomatic disorders, is uttered in *The Scarlet Letter* by the scholarly physician Roger Chillingworth about the "rare case" (135) of pastor Arthur Dimmesdale, whose mysteriously declining health puzzles and intrigues him. "A bodily disease," Chillingworth explains to Dimmesdale, "which we look upon as whole and entire in itself, may, after all, be but a symptom of some ailment in the spiritual part" (135). The connection that Chillingworth here makes between the physical and the psychological seems at first glance anachronistically modern in a work published in 1850, yet actually it is in consonance with the premodern holistic conceptions of humoral medicine. The action of *The Scarlet Letter* takes place "not less than two centuries" (57) previous to 1850, at a time when the close conjunction of body and mind was an integral facet of the prevailing belief system. According to humoral medicine, the "sympathy betwixt soul and body" would in fact have been the natural expectation rather than a "strange" phenomenon.

Apart from the medical theories of the mid-seventeenth century, Hawthorne could also have drawn on his own recent personal experience. In 1849, at the age of forty-five, Hawthorne lost the job he had held for three years at the Salem Custom House. His position was precarious for he had not yet sufficiently established his reputation as a writer to be able to support his family by the pen alone. A few weeks later his mother died. In the aftermath of this double loss, Hawthorne sickened. The writing of *The Scarlet Letter* later that summer can be seen not only as a means to earn money but also as a form of therapy. When Hawthorne read the story's final pages to his wife in February 1850, he reports that it broke her heart and sent her to bed with "a grievous headache." This little incident might have confirmed for Hawthorne the potential that distressing emotions have for conversion into physical symptoms.

In *The Scarlet Letter* the social context is of such decisive importance that any reading must begin on this "intervening variable."[1] Its crucial momentum is indicated by the fact that the narrative opens on a description of the environment. The novel, which has been designated as "the single indispensable study of Puritan culture,"[2] rests entirely on that culture's premises and beliefs. The Massachusetts Bay colony was in many ways eclectic, even in its unusual legal structure as a business corporation chartered with authority to exert jurisdiction over the lands it occupied. The main purpose of the Puritan experiment in its early days was "to show that men could govern themselves in a political state exactly as they governed themselves in a church organization."[3] The original settlers intended to base their legal system almost exclusively on biblical authority, but in practice this proved awkward in the judgment of ordinary civil and criminal cases.

Establishment of the Bible as a legal code had the effect of elevating clerical opinion to unprecedented heights. Ministers ruled on most legal issues; acting in their capacity as accredited biblical scholars, they were invested with final moral authority in civil as well as spiritual matters. If the New England colony was "a city on a hill,"[4] its clergy were "the bright and shining Lights" in the "golden Candlesticks.[5] For the figure of Dimmesdale in *The Scarlet Letter* it is vital to understand this extraordinary exaltation of ministers, who wielded immense power by playing a lead part in determining who among the settlers had experienced a true conversion and so deserved the privilege of franchise.

The "early severity of the Puritan character" (57) in the new colony is underscored from the outset of *The Scarlet Letter*. The title of the first chapter, "The Prison Door," immediately indicates the shortfall in the settlement's utopian aspirations to virtue and happiness, for space had already had to be allotted not only to a cemetery but also to a prison. Of these two, the cemetery is, despite its finality, the less unpalatable because it is merely the completion of the normal course of human life whereas the prison is a place of punishment for violations of the colony's laws. The very necessity for a prison thus represents a transgressive infraction of the Puritans' religiously inspired ideals. The scene in the second section, "The Market Place," where Hester is put into the pillory, shows "the grim rigidity" (57) typical of this milieu, where religion and law are "almost identical" (58). The harsh ethos of this time and place is conveyed in a series of attendant factors: the existence of a scaffold as "a portion of a penal machine" (62), regarded as "an agent in the promotion of good citizenship" (62–63); the virtually uniform virulence of the female spectators in their condemnation of Hester, and "the grim beadle" who pronounces "a blessing on the righteous Colony of the Massachusetts, where iniquity is dragged out into the sunshine!" (62). The fundamentalist vindictiveness evident in these reactions to Hester creates an ominous atmosphere for the whole narrative, and the sense of apprehension is heightened by Hawthorne's tactic of giving initially only hints about the nature of "the taint of deepest sin" (63) of which Hester had been found guilty.

The presentation of this Puritan milieu also reveals a central feature of the literary strategy of *The Scarlet Letter:* the repeated resonance of the figurative within the literal. The narrative is rich in descriptive details, all of which carry dismal connotations. In the opening sentence, the throng of bearded men wear "sad-colored garments" (55); there are "iron spikes" (55) on the prison door; the "weather stains and other indications of age gave a yet darker aspect to its beetle-browed and gloomy front" (55); the "unsightly," "overgrown" (56) vegetation about the prison is described as "the black flower of civilized society" (56). This somber surface suggests the grim, cramped environment established by the Puritans. The pressure of group standards on the nonconforming individual is extremely strong. Yet a single object of beauty still flourishes, the rosebush by the prison entrance that has somehow "survived out of the stern old wilderness" (56) and that even bears flowers. Its metaphoric implications are clearly spelled out by the narrator: "It may serve, let us hope, to symbolize some sweet moral blossom that may be found along the track, or relieve the darkening close of a tale of human frailty and sorrow" (56).

Such imbrication of the figurative within the literal is even more prominent in the colony's relationship to its surroundings. The marketplace, the primary forum of the Puritans' activities, is throughout contrasted with the forest on its perimeter. The forest's intrinsically heathen nature is first intimated by its role as the home of the native Indians, one of whom stands on the outskirts of the crowd at the pillory. The settlers are therefore threatened not only by transgressors within their community but also by their possibly hostile outer environment. So the colony itself is a confine, an enclosure turned in on itself, deliberately cut off from the flow of life natural to the forest. The Puritans' self-imposed opposition to both the old world that they had left and the new in which they are embedded is a likely source of tension through their programmatic isolation in their cult of virtue.

In Hester's mind, the forest is the incarnation of "the moral wilderness in which she had so long been wandering" (175). It is in the forest that Pearl, the offspring of adultery, cavorts at her pleasure; Chillingworth roams the forest to gather herbs and to spy; Hester meets Dimmesdale there, and there too she, Dimmesdale, and Pearl can be a united family. "We must not always talk in the market place of what happens to us in the forest" (225), Hester explains to Pearl, making clear to the child the divergent codes that govern the two adjacent spheres. The forest close by the market place is dangerous, amoral, proliferating in accordance with its unfettered nature, the alluring counteragent to the Puritans' restrictive standards. The symbolic charge of the forest as the antithesis to religiousness is unmistakably implicit in Mistress Hibbins's taunt of Dimmesdale: "Who, now, that saw him pass in the procession, would think how little while it is since he went forth out of his study—chewing a Hebrew text of Scripture in his mouth, I warrant—to take an airing in the forest!" (226)

Mistress Hibbins, "the reputed witch-lady" (208), is a further strand in the social context of *The Scarlet Letter*. For the Puritans' religiousness is shown to be rife with superstition. In addition to the recognizable external menace of the forest and the overt internal one of transgressors, the Puritans have an acute fear of more subtle subversion by hidden evil lurking everywhere in their midst. For instance, instead of grass, black weeds grow on the grave of a man thought to have died an unconfessed sinner. Meteors and other natural phenomena are interpreted "as so many revelations from a supernatural source" (150). Dimmesdale thinks he sees "an immense letter—the letter 'A'—marked out in lines of dull red light" (151) in the sky. On his return from the forest, he fully expects to find "an evil spirit" (210) in his study. Most commonly, as on this occasion, it is Chillingworth who is identified as that evil spirit; Hester inquires, half-teasingly, whether he is "like the Black Man that haunts the forest round about us" (81). So the heathenness of the forest is connected to both the blackness of sin and the prevalence of superstition. At Dimmesdale's last sermon, Chillingworth, looking "dark, disturbed, and evil," "rose up out of some nether region" (225). Dimmesdale, too, is associated with "Satan" when he encounters a pure, newly converted young woman, and "the archfiend whispered him to condense into small compass and drop into her tender bosom a germ of evil that would be sure to blossom darkly soon, and bear black fruit betimes" (207). Indeed, Mistress Hibbins asks Dimmesdale directly whether he has sold himself "to the fiend" (209). Hester herself is usually left to stand in "a small vacant area—a sort of magic circle" (220), while Pearl, because of her mischievous exuberance as well as her illegitimate birth, is widely considered a "witch-baby" (229). Thus the superstition that accompanies religion spawns an undertow of anxiety among the colonists.

This atmosphere of tension, superstition, suspicion, and intolerance fosters concealment of any putative breach of the Puritans' severe code of behavior. Since they believed that "transgressions deserve punishment,"[6] immediate retribution was meted out in public together with continued social ostracism, as the case of Hester illustrates. Only in the forest is there "no peril of discovery" (143), and even there Chillingworth stalks wrong-doers. However, at this remove from the jurisdiction and influence of the colony, Dimmesdale is able, at least temporarily, to shed "all the dread of public exposure that had so long been the anguish of his life" (148). Repression and denial are shown to be almost inevitable consequences of a righteousness taken to terrorist extremes. Such a societal order is conducive to the development of psychosomatic disorders as an avenue of escape, a culturally sanctioned means to avoid a distressing impasse.

Ironically, in *The Scarlet Letter* Dimmesdale's illness is condoned because it is misinterpreted. His failing health, a major motif in the narrative, is ultimately more of "a riddle" (68) than the paternity of Hester's child. The two occurrences, the baby's birth and the beginning of Dimmesdale's decline, are linked casually, not causally, in a parishioner's early comment: "[T]he Reverend Master Dimmesdale, her [Hester's] godly pastor, takes it very grievously to heart that such a scandal should have come upon his congregation" (59). In the public view, his grief springs from his sense of responsibility for the congregationists under his spiritual care. Taking something to heart is a very apposite phrase in this context, for it is applicable to soul and body alike. Dimmesdale's frequent gesture of holding his hand to his heart, noticed by everyone around him, is left open to alternative readings. Does he actually experience a physical sensation of pain or discomfort such as could denote heart disease? Or does his habit of reaching for his heart have a primarily psychological connotation as an unvoiced expression of distress?

Dimmesdale's symptoms are vague and diffuse in a manner often characteristic of psychosomatic disorders. He himself never mentions any complaints, although this disregard is in keeping with the stoicism befitting a Puritan minister. His taciturnity may be innate to his personality, but as no information is given about his background, formation, or earlier career, there are no grounds for assessing his current silence. His tenacious resistance to speaking out is, of course, a means to evade detection, yet it is also a cardinal factor in the etiology of the conversion of his psychological pain into physical manifestations. So Dimmesdale's reticence, while socially approved, is undoubtedly damaging to his well-being. If he is fulfilling the regimen of self-examination by which the repentant sinner, according to the Puritan doctrine of preparation, could estimate his readiness for receiving grace, this exercise could increase his anxiety "because it transferred authority over the self to the self."[7] So Dimmesdale can only turn in on himself. In the environment in which he lives and especially in the position he occupies, he has no one to whom he could legitimately speak, especially in view of the nature of his transgression. His function, after all, is that of recipient of confessions, the keeper of the communal conscience. Dimmesdale's professional role reinforces the social pressure on him. Discretion blends with fear to hold him in check.

The changes in Dimmesdale are recorded through his parishioners' observations and the narrator's notations. For instance, it is stated that the young minister's "health had severely suffered of late" (109); that "about this period, . . . the health of Mr. Dimmesdale had evidently begun to fail" (119). The temporal indicator ("about this period") points to the coincidence of the beginning of Dimmesdale's decline with the intense stress occasioned by the scandal in his congregation. Hester notices his pallor and his custom of "holding his hand over his heart . . . whenever his peculiarly nervous temperament was thrown into agitation" (113). Here the physical gesture is linked to his state of mind ("agitation"), although the causal connection remains a matter of conjecture. The narrator, while asserting that Dimmesdale "looked now more careworn and emaciated than we described him at the scene of Hester's public ignominy," leaves open the possibilities he raises: "[W]hether it were his failing health, or whatever the cause might be, his large dark eyes had a world of pain in their troubled and melancholy depth" (113). Chillingworth, his physician, meditates on Dimmesdale's "strange reserve," on the fact that "the nature of Mr. Dimmesdale's bodily disease had never fairly been revealed to him" (123). Increasingly, Dimmesdale is in the grip of "the gnawing and poisonous tooth of bodily pain" (144). Hester is "shocked at the condition to which she found the clergyman reduced" (154). He comes to look "haggard and feeble" (179), with "a listlessness in his gait" and "a nerveless despondency in his air" (180). The hypothesis that his symptoms are psychosomatic in origin is supported by the brief upsurge of strength he experiences with the dawn of hope when Hester persuades him to leave the colony to start a new life together in England. The mere prospect of release from his oppressive environment raises his spirits and instils some energy into him. But mostly he is portrayed as "suffering under bodily disease, and gnawed and tortured by some black trouble of the soul" (138). The interplay of body and soul is clearly articulated in the striking image of the emotional trouble *eating* into the body like some predatory vermin.

Dimmesdale aggravates his state by the extremism of the religious devotions he imposes on himself. To readers who already suspect his role in Hester's disgrace his excesses signal attempts at self-chastisement and penitence. But to his wholly unsuspecting parishioners Dimmesdale's behavior appears on the contrary an indication of his heightened virtue. They attribute his failing health to "his too unreserved self-sacrifice to the labors and duties of the pastoral relation" (109). They radically misread his stance: "By those best acquainted with his habits, the paleness of the young minister's cheek was accounted for by his too earnest devotion to study, his scrupulous fulfillment of parochial duty, and, more than all, by the fasts and vigils of which he made a frequent practice, in order to keep the grossness of this earthly state from clogging and obscuring his spiritual lamp" (119). They are so convinced of his holiness that they believe that if he were to die, it would be because "the world was not worthy to be any longer trodden by his feet" (119). A rumor spreads that the advent of an eminent physician to the colony is "an absolute miracle" (120) wrought by heaven to save Dimmesdale. The irony of these misinterpretations is hinted in the rhetoric of overstatement the narrator ascribes to the parishioners, who see Chillingworth as having been bodily transported through the air and set "down at the door of Mr. Dimmesdale's study" (120). Through the reiterated use of indirect discourse Hawthorne is able, without authorial comment, to uncover the sharp dichotomy between the colonists' perceptions of Dimmesdale and readers' growing surmise of the very different motivation of his bizarre conduct.

As a result of the widespread misunderstanding of the situation, the esteem in which Dimmesdale is held rises in proportion to his increasing physical debility. Dimmesdale's self-castigation is misread as a sign of his advance toward sainthood. The fragility of his "frame" (139), by making him seem ethereal, intensifies his "fame"; he is deemed "a miracle of holiness" (139) at the very time when he himself questions whether grass will ever grow on his grave "because an accursed thing must there be buried!" (139). His "emaciated figure, his thin cheek, his white, heavy, pain-wrinkled brow" elicit "deep, almost worshipping respect" (205). The emphasis is always on the discrepancy between the public homage and his corporeal infirmity, which is mistaken as evidence of his sanctity. At his "very proudest eminence" (232), when he preaches his last, stirring sermon on a holiday, the listeners speculate: "Were there not the brilliant particles of a halo about his head?" (233). Dimmesdale reaches the zenith of veneration simultaneously with the nadir of his enfeeblement. This disparity lends a neat structural chiasmus to *The Scarlet Letter* as well as a persistent undercurrent of irony.

The imminence of Dimmesdale's death is mentioned so often that it hardly comes as a surprise. Aesthetically it is the only appropriate closure to this "tale of human frailty and sorrow" (56); it would contravene the entire moral thrust of the story to have Dimmesdale and Hester leave for England on the presumption that they could there live happily ever after. In the Puritan system sinners cannot reap happiness. No medical explanation of his sudden death is offered; such unexplained deaths were not unusual in the mid-seventeenth century. Dimmesdale's death is a logical necessity in the context of the Puritan belief that the wages of sin were death and damnation.

So does Dimmesdale succumb to heart disease? That is a possibility, in light of the overload of stress under which he has been laboring. While psychosomatic disorders are not in themselves fatal, "eventual diagnosis of a general medical condition . . . is frequent."[8] The physical diagnosis of Dimmesdale's death is secondary to its figurative import. Like the scarlet letter itself, all the elements in the narrative are suffused with a pronounced metaphoricity, with the result that they lend themselves to interpretation on both a realistic and a figurative plane. Dimmesdale's illness and death are prime examples of the symbolizing mode of narration that gives *The Scarlet Letter* such remarkable density and power.

In the portrayal of Chillingworth an equally clear correlation becomes apparent between the figurative and the literal in his changing appearance. Chillingworth is first characterized in Hester's memory of him as "the misshapen scholar" (66). Through this "slight deformity" (67) Hester recognizes him when he appears on the edge of the crowd in the marketplace, standing, significantly next to an Indian from the forest. Chillingworth's physical deficit consists of an asymmetry that is the cipher for his emotional imbalance. Hester herself, in her flashback of her life as she stands in the pillory, visualizes Chillingworth as "a man well stricken in years, a pale, thin, scholar-like visage" (65), but she recalls nothing of the circumstances that led to the union of this incongruent pair. For his part, Chillingworth, in his interview with Hester in the prison, where he is admitted in his capacity as a physician, is quite open in assuming the blame for what he terms his "folly": "Misshapen from my birth-hour, how could I delude myself with the idea that intellectual gifts might veil physical deformity in a young girl's fantasy!" (78). When Hester murmurs "I have greatly wronged thee," he responds: "We have wronged each other" (79). In his visit to Hester, Chillingworth appears in a favorable light, showing both honesty and generosity. Yet his solicitude for her, mingled perhaps with a residual conjugal possessiveness, leads to his obsession with ferreting out the man "who has wronged us both!" (79). "He will be known!" (69), he vows thrice in succession. In another emphatic repetition, Chillingworth's pledge, "Sooner or later, he must needs be mine!" is heightened into the even stronger, "[H]e shall be mine!" (80). As he becomes ever more consumed by his determination to pursue the wrongdoer by every means, Chillingworth grows increasingly sinister in body as much as in spirit. Hester is "startled to perceive what a change had come over his features—how much uglier they were—how his dark complexion seemed to have grown duskier, and his figure more misshapen" (112). She is shocked at the change in him over the years, not so much at the signs of advancing age as at "his blackness" that he can no longer mask (163). The physical transformation that Hester sees represents the external figuration of Chillingworth's emotional state, another instance, as in Dimmesdale's case, of the "strange sympathy betwixt soul and body".

The reciprocal impact of Dimmesdale and Chillingworth on each other becomes the main focus of interest in *The Scarlet Letter*. Hester, in the forefront at the beginning, recedes as she settles into a modest existence as a needlewoman. The narrative is punctuated by sections that trace her progress, but her consistent refusal to disclose her secret makes her relatively static psychologically. On the other hand, Dimmesdale—who is so peripheral a figure in the first third of *The Scarlet Letter* that when he reappears Hawthorne introduces him once more as "the Reverend Arthur Dimmesdale, whom the reader may remember as having taken a brief and reluctant part in the scene of Hester's disgrace" (109)—slowly moves from being so marginal as to be forgettable to center stage. Chillingworth, too, comes to attract increasing attention, entering the forum of the action through his professional standing as a physician. The call to attend to the baby Pearl is the plot device that facilitates the private interview with Hester, the occasion for revealing their status as "a married pair" (79). Chillingworth's subsequent attendance on Dimmesdale is the catalyst to the cardinal psychodynamic interaction in *The Scarlet Letter*. Chillingworth's enterprise is that of a detective intent on finding the perpetrator of the crime, but his methods also derive from those of a psychiatrist aiming to elicit the etiology of a disorder.

The trigger to Dimmesdale's disintegration is transparent once the plot unfolds: his deep sense of guilt about his seduction of Hester and his faithlessness to her. In the context of Puritanism, Dimmesdale's act is not merely a human lapse but a betrayal of his mission. Dimmesdale's name suggests the split in him; his first name, Arthur, evokes romance through its association with Arthurian romance. His last name, however, sends a different message: "dim" is self-explanatory, and "dale" has its etymology in something bent or bending, a hollow, low ground between hills. The pastor's behavior toward Hester is certainly bent, as well as hollow in his betrayal of her trust by not publicly standing by her. What is more, as Chillingworth realizes, Dimmesdale, "pure as they deem him—all spiritual as he seems—hath inherited a strong animal nature from his father or his mother" (128). Hester, for her part, is described as being "of an impulsive and passionate nature" (64). These apparently stray comments underpin their encounter(s) which, we guess, probably took place in the forest.

Dimmesdale's recognition of the multiple betrayals he has committed toward Hester, toward his professional obligations, toward his religious creed is at the root of his affliction. At his first appearance already there are signs of his profound malaise; he has "an apprehensive, a startled, a half-frightened look—of a being who felt himself quite astray and at a loss in the pathway of human existence" (72). His egoistical, self-protective silence places him in a dire position since his charge is to "deal with this poor sinner's [Hester's] soul" (71). Dimmesdale is neither inarticulate nor lacking in self-awareness; his silence is purely a means of self-defense, and his understanding of his own stance must intensify his distress. His appreciation of the "wondrous strength and generosity of a woman's heart" (74) in upholding her—their—secret intensifies his shame at his own cowardice. So he is weighed down by a twin load of guilt, for his original transgression and for his subsequent pusillanimity. He pleads, successfully, to the colony's governor for Hester to be allowed to keep Pearl when the Puritans think her unfit to bring a child up in the proper manner. Dimmesdale argues that having the opportunity to guide the child along the right path makes "the sinful mother happier than the sinful father" (114). The repetition of the word "sinful" shows that he conceives his lapse in a religious light as "sinful" rather than under the civil aspect of responsibility or from the humane angle as loyalty. His internalization of the public values of his community creates severe intrapsychic conflicts. As "a religion of self-scrutiny," Puritanism encouraged its members to turn "inward with merciless demands on the self, . . . rooting out their own deviants in their midst."[9]

The mental suffering that springs internally from Dimmesdale's conscience is vastly exacerbated by Chillingworth's intervention. How Chillingworth comes to identify Dimmesdale as the perpetrator of the dastardly deed is, like much else in *The Scarlet Letter*, merely hinted. The "godly pastor" (59) is, after all, the least likely culprit. Chillingworth's suspicions are first aroused during the scene at the governor's palace when Dimmesdale's impassioned plea thwarts the attempt to remove Pearl from Hester. His plea, together with Pearl's behavior, alerts Chillingworth to the possibility of their relatedness. Having refused to go near the Reverend Mr. Wilson, Pearl takes Dimmesdale's hand, and after an instant of hesitation, he responds by kissing her brow. The incident is so slight compared to the issue of guardianship that the reader may overlook it. Not so Chillingworth's practiced eye as a physician: "Would it be beyond a philosopher's research, . . . to analyze the child's nature, and, from its make and mould, to give a shrewd guess at the father?" (115).

Cannily, though with seeming innocence, Chillingworth establishes a connection to Dimmesdale by choosing him to be "his spiritual guide" (119). As the minister's health begins to falter, he is urged by his parishioners to "make trial of the physician's frankly offered skill," an offer that Dimmesdale at first rejects peremptorily: "I need no medicine" (120). Still, Chillingworth insinuates himself into Dimmesdale's life, becoming a lodger in the same house as well as his medical adviser. The interest the two develop in each other is mutual; indeed, as "a deep intimacy" (123) grows between them, their entire rapport is similar to transference and countertransference in psychotherapy. Taking long walks together for the sake of Dimmesdale's health, they engage in "various talk" (121). Dimmesdale feels "a fascination" for "the man of science" whose "intellectual cultivation" (123) opens up a whole range of new ideas to him. "It was as if a window were thrown open, admitting a freer atmosphere into the close and stifled study where his life was wasting away. . . . But the air was too fresh and chill to be long breathed with comfort" (122). The image of the window thrown open suggests the new insights afforded by psychotherapy, while the excessive chill of the air alludes to Dimmesdale's discomfort with the knowledge he has to confront.

If Dimmesdale is wary of Chillingworth, the "anxious and attached physician" (123) has a highly complicated countertransference to his patient, for his intention is to exploit a legitimate medical relationship for the ulterior purpose of extracting revenge. He is puzzled by Dimmesdale's condition; in a manner characteristic of psychosomatic disorders, the physician faces a quandary: "[T]he disease is what I seem to know, yet know it not" (133). Fully cognizant of the "strange sympathy betwixt soul and body" (135), Chillingworth is "strongly moved to look into the character and qualities of the patient" (121) as an integral facet of his disease. For he deems it essential "to know the man before attempting to do him good. Whenever there is a heart and an intellect, the diseases of the physical frame are tinged with the peculiarities of these" (122). In the temporal context of *The Scarlet Letter* this approach can be ascribed to humoral medicine's belief in patient-specific treatment, but it also shows genuine insight into psychosomatic disorders in the acknowledgment of the role of emotions in bodily complaints. Trying to discover the sources of Dimmesdale's disorder, Chillingworth explains to him that "a sore place, if we may so call it, in your spirit hath immediately its appropriate manifestation in your bodily frame" (134). Here again the inseparability of mind and body is emphasized, as well as the likelihood that it is a psychological disturbance that is surfacing in a physical guise. In Dimmesdale Chillingworth sees, as he tells him, "of all men whom I have known, [the one] whose body is the closest conjoined, and imbued, and identified, so to speak, with the spirit whereof it is the instrument" (133). This trenchant formulation of the etiology of a psychosomatic disorder alarms Dimmesdale precisely because it is on target. He hastily dismisses Chillingworth with the ironic rejoinder: "You deal not, I take it, in medicine for the soul" (133).

Chillingworth actually dispenses antimedicine, or poison, for Dimmesdale's soul. The particle "Chill" in his name (and as an adjective that could qualify the air let into the window of Dimmesdale's study) projects the coldness of his calculation in regard to his patient. He is also referred to in *The Scarlet Letter* as "the leech,"—an ambiguous term, since leeches were much used up to the mid-nineteenth century as therapeutic agents, yet the drawing of blood could result in the weakening and even death of the patient. Chillingworth's leech-like quality resides in his infiltration into Dimmesdale's life and psyche as a malevolent force. He gnaws and consumes his quarry with at least as much venom as the minister's conscience, his internal devil; he becomes the extraneous "devil" (163), the catalyst to Dimmesdale's collapse. The images applied to him underline the relentlessness of his burrowing on his sinister mission: he is "like a treasure-seeker in a dark cavern" (122), digging "into the poor clergyman's heart like a miner searching for gold; or, rather, like a sexton delving into a grave, possibly in quest of a jewel that had been buried on the dead man's bosom, but likely to find nothing save mortality and corruption" (127). The destructiveness of this antitherapeutic process, in which Chillingworth devotes seven years "to the constant analysis of a heart" (164), makes him as much of a perversion of the medical profession as Dimmesdale is of the clergy. Both are supposed to be concerned with the care of souls, and each in his own way is a parodistic inversion of the ideal.

In hunting the culprit down, Chillingworth himself becomes a criminal, when he gives Dimmesdale a draught that plunges him into a deep sleep. What Chillingworth glimpses on the drugged clergyman's chest is left to readers' imagination, stimulated by the information that "a wild look of wonder, joy and horror . . . a ghastly rapture" bursts "through the whole ugliness of his figure" (135). After this incident their relationship changes, with "a quiet depth of malice, hitherto latent, but active now" on the physician's part, and a "shy and sensitive reserve" (136), that is, a resisting withdrawal on Dimmesdale's side. The former "deep intimacy" (123) is transformed into "a more intimate revenge than any mortal had ever wreaked upon an enemy" (136). Chillingworth becomes "not a spectator only, but a chief actor in the poor minister's interior world" (137). Dimmesdale is also described as "the victim forever on the rack" once the physician knows "the spring that controlled the engine" (137). Dimmesdale has "constantly a dim awareness of some evil influence watching over him" (137). Under the pressure of "the machinations of his deadliest enemy" (138), he disintegrates completely. Outwardly still a "subtile but remorseful hypocrite" (140), his "constant introspection" (141) effects torture without purification. Both Chillingworth and Dimmesdale act by intuition, nurturing reciprocal suspicion, yet denied definitive confirmation. This limbo of semicertainty impells Chillingworth to ever greater cruelty until Dimmesdale in a crisis compounded of guilt, fear, terrible anxiety, shame, intense misery, and acute self-loathing wonders whether he is "going mad" (146). Hester, too, sees him "on the verge of lunacy" (160), but she understands both the origins of his physical and mental decompensation and Chillingworth's nefarious role in precipitating it. If Chillingworth is associated with "a snake" (67), the repressed secret itself is "like a serpent" (84) rising from its hole.

The latent presence of secrets is a key theme in *The Scarlet Letter;* the word itself recurs countless times. Indeed, a psychologist has summarized the novel as showing "how a pathogenic secret can be discovered by a wicked man and exploited in order to torture his victim to death."[10] Each of the three main protagonists guards a secret, and in two instances it proves pathogenic.

The exception is Hester, although her secret forms the crux of the story. Her expulsion from the community has severe repercussions for her socially and spiritually, for in Puritanism "the key idea of the new theology was that an individual's relationship to God needed to be screened by some intermediate level of authority—a congregation, a government, an administration."[11] Exclusion from the community thus diminishes hopes of ultimate salvation. Yet, ironically, Hester conforms to the ideal if New England is perceived "as a colony of heroic sufferers."[12] Curiously unscathed psychologically, and seemingly uncowed by Puritan teachings, she is free of conflicts, and therefore physically and psychologically healthy. Unlike Dimmesdale, she is "not afraid of nightmares and hideous dreams" (81). In her stoical acceptance of her guilt and her capacity to rebuild her life on a sound, though limited basis, she is an idealized figure. Hester avoids the potential damage of her secret by not turning inward onto herself into a downward spiral of self-incrimination. She is not wholly free of burden, for "she grew pale whenever it [the secret] struggled from her heart" (84).

However, she derives strength, purpose in life, and eventually even social respect from looking outward to help others. Instead of fleeing, as people had expected, she settles in an abandoned cottage on the outskirts of the town, not in close proximity to any other house so that her home's "comparative remoteness" (84) places her beyond the immediate sphere of social activity. This location is the embodiment of Hester's liminality, and her choice of this abode denotes her understanding of and assent to her marginal position. The obligation to care for her child and to earn a living proves salutary too in mobilizing her energy into positive channels and to attainable goals. By her dignity and her fine work as a needlewoman Hester earns grudging admiration. Above all, through the role she assumes "as a self-enlisted Sister of Charity" (203), she both redeems herself morally and regains a social function on the perimeter of the community. Such good works were not considered efficacious in themselves, but the Puritans held the "conviction that the acts of the outward person can be used as a gauge, albeit an imperfect one, to the inner person."[13]

Besides the paternity of her child, Hester has a second secret almost more painful to her, "the secret bond" (89) between herself and Chillingworth. This second secret gives *The Scarlet Letter* its structural symmetry: the bearer of the scarlet letter is tied by hidden links to the two men who flank her and who play out the central struggle in the narrative. Hester's yielding to Dimmesdale can be seen as a spontaneous expression of her "impulsive and passionate nature" (64), a result of her loneliness, and a response to his attractiveness as a young man held in high esteem in the colony. Her prior marriage to Chillingworth is harder to explain, is in fact not explained, except as an outcome of Chillingworth's "folly" (79). This second secret weighs more heavily on Hester than that represented by the scarlet letter, probably because she cannot fathom her deed vis-à-vis Chillingworth as she can that with Dimmesdale. Her avowal to Dimmesdale of her relationship to Chillingworth, at a late stage in the story, is replete with shame and anger: "That old man!—the physician!—he whom they call Roger Chillingworth!—he was my husband!" (184). Nonetheless, in the face of Dimmesdale's horror and refusal to forgive, Hester still stands firm. Whatever her past, she maintains a fundamental integrity that assures her mental health. A major difference between Hester and the two other holders of secrets in *The Scarlet Letter* lies in her persistent silence as much, or more, to protect others rather than herself. A connection to either Dimmesdale or Chillingworth would be advantageous to Hester, though damaging to them. This streak of altruism distinguishes her from the two men.

In contrast, Dimmesdale is the one most plagued by his secret because it forces him into a position of inauthenticity, alienating him from his professional calling as well as from his inner self. For this reason his secret becomes pathogenic in a way that Hester's does not for her. He, too, has given in to a normal drive of his "strong animal nature" (128), doing "a wild thing . . . this pious Master Dimmesdale, in the hot passion of his heart" (134). By keeping his secret hidden, Dimmesdale forfeits his self-respect in addition to his peace of mind. He comes to hate himself as "a pollution and a lie" on account of "the black secret in his soul" (140). The Puritans saw "sin as excrescence, disease—the threatening other—against which the community of purist selves builds barricades."[14] The Puritans' equation of sin with disease is of utmost importance for Dimmesdale. His guilt is further intensified by his parishioners' misinterpretation of his fasts and vigils—and his physical decline—as signs of a growing holiness. The discrepancy between his reputation and his reality is a source of torment to him as an ever falser image is projected onto him by the community. He knows well enough that the "[r]emorse which dogged him everywhere" is held in check by "[c]owardice which invariably drew him back with her tremulous grip" (144). Even Pearl reproaches him: "Thou warst not bold!—thou warst not true!" (152). Unable either to cope with his secret or to dissociate himself from it, Dimmesdale unconsciously converts it into tangible, visible symptoms as an overt idiom of distress over which he has no control. While his choices in the moral sphere may be unpalatable, at least he does have some choice, although he lacks the courage to exercise it. But the "sore" that Dimmesdale manages more or less to "hide" (133) as long as it remains in his soul, cannot be contained once the conversion into bodily disorders sets in. The confluence of soul and body takes place symbolically in the heart, which is both a corporeal organ and a spiritual entity. "What is it that the minister seeks to hide with his hand always over his heart?" (227), Mistress Hibbins asks Hester. Through the reiterated gesture of holding his hand over his heart, Dimmesdale simultaneously conceals and reveals. It is an involuntary gesture that signifies his conflicted need for secrecy and avoidance on the one hand, and on the other for oblique, furtive disclosure as a form of confession. For Dimmesdale is so "overwhelmed with shame" (147) that, short of going mad, as he fears, has has to find an outlet of some kind, and that outlet takes the form of a conversion disorder.

As Dimmesdale exhibits increasingly visible symptoms of physical illness, he is pressed by his parishioners into the physician's hands. Chillingworth is the most enigmatic figure in *The Scarlet Letter*; he is described as "the mysterious old Roger Chillingworth" (121), and even his name is an "appellation" (117) that he chooses to use in the colony. His past in Europe and as Hester's husband is sketched only vaguely, so that he is veiled by disguise and narratorial reticence. It is solely his scientific expertise that validates him: "He was heard to speak of Sir Kenelm Digby, and other famous men— . . . as having been his correspondents or associates. Why, with such rank in the learned world, had he come hither? What could he, whose sphere was in great cities, be seeking in the wilderness?" (120) The questions remain unanswered: Has Chillingworth come to reclaim his wife? If so, how had they been parted? Had Hester fled him to the new world to which he follows in pursuit? Himself shrouded in mystery, Chillingworth is drawn to the "riddle" (68) posed by Hester's obdurate discretion. In addition to his strong personal interest in Hester, Chillingworth has the innate curiosity of the scholar-scientist, the urge to attain knowledge and mastery. Professionally also, as a physician to soul and body, he is accustomed to deciphering puzzles. So he boasts to Hester, "[T]here are few things—whether in the outward world, or to a certain depth, in the invisible sphere of thought—few things hidden from the man who devotes himself earnestly and unreservedly to the solution of a mystery" (79).

Chillingworth's natural inclination to probe a mystery, especially one that concerns the paternity of his wife's child, is perverted by his thirst for revenge. He deviates from merely wanting to solve a problem to an obsession with vengeance once his suspicions fall on Dimmesdale. The challenge shifts from simple detection to the psychological manipulation of the wrongdoer. Chillingworth's aim is less to induce Dimmesdale to confess his sin than to undo him completely by a process of sustained demoralization. Under the pretense of medical assistance and friendship, Chillingworth acts out his obsession at his own expense as well as Dimmesdale's. He therefore becomes the keeper of two secrets: Dimmesdale's and his own. His is more complex than the minister's, which centers on a single misdeed for which he feels a mixture of "guilt and sorrow" (228). If Dimmesdale is not prepared to risk a public declaration and the catastrophic disgrace and punishment such an act would entail, he is at least open to Hester's suggestion that they leave for England; he thereby shows his willingness to make amends to her and to Pearl—provided this, too, can be done under the cover of secrecy. Chillingworth's secret, on the other hand, is more heinous insofar as it is motivated by jealously, rancor, and malice. While Dimmesdale is driven by the urge to protect himself, Chllingworth sets out in a calculated manner to injure another. In terms of this Puritan society, he is doing the "Devil's work" for the "very principle" of his life is said "to consist in the pursuit and systematic exercise of revenge" (242). But his secret takes its toll—its own revenge, as it were—on him in a rebound effect; he is progressively tranformed into a darker, uglier figure, and ultimately consumed by a passion fiercer and certainly more pernicious than Dimmesdale's.

Readers, too, are sucked into the web of secrecy in *The Scarlet Letter,* for it does not have the informational plenitude and specificity customary in mid-nineteenth-century narrative. Large gaps abound not only about Chillingworth but also about the past of both Hester and Dimmesdale. The characters appear almost out of nowhere, enact the drama, and fade from sight. A striking example of a lacuna of uncertainty is the unresolved question as to what Chillingworth glimpses on Dimmesdale's chest while the minister is in a drugged sleep. The physician's "rapture" at whatever he espies is "too mighty to be expressed only by the eye and features, and therefore bursting through the whole ugliness of his figure, and making itself even riotously manifest by the extravagant gestures with which he threw his arms towards the ceiling, and stamped his foot upon the floor!" (135). Like Dimmesdale holding his hand over his heart, Chillingworth here expresses his feelings not in words but in physical gestures that parallel the process of conversion. Readers surmise that there is actually a scarlet letter inscribed on Dimmesdale's body. "Mother," Pearl exclaims, "he has his hand over his heart! Is it because, when the minister wrote his name in the book, the Black Man set his mark in that place? But why does he not wear it outside his bosom, as thou dost?" (179). Is the mark to be read literally or figuratively? At the hour of his death Dimmesdale addresses his parishioners: "He bids you look again at Hester's scarlet letter! He tells you that, with all its mysterious horror, it is but the shadow of what he bears on his own breast, and that even this, his own red stigma, is not more than the type of what has seared his own heart!" (238). He tears away his clothing: "It was revealed! But it were irreverent to describe that revelation. For an instant, the gaze of the horror-stricken multitude was concentred on the ghastly miracle" (238). With consummate skill Hawthorne shifts the decision onto the reactions of witnesses—and how reliable are they, imbued as they are with superstition and readily amenable to suggestion? The onus of ultimate choice is thus imposed on readers who are made aware of a secret and left to reach their own conclusions, like the colonists.

The narrator is also embroiled in this web of secrecy. Sometimes he makes an open appearance, invoking readers' assent by the plural "we," but he is far from omniscient. He resorts to the subterfuge, popular in romantic literature, of his own dependence on "a manuscript of old date, drawn up from the verbal testimony of individuals, some of whom had known Hester Prynne, while others had heard the tale from contemporary witnesses" (241). The narrator designates this manuscript as "the authority which we have chiefly followed" and claims that it "fully confirms the view taken in the foregoing pages" (242). This overarching frame casts an aura of uncertainty over the entire narrative; its origins are as obscure as those of its main figures, and its alleged "authority" derives from "contemporary witnesses," some of whom had known Hester while others had merely "heard the tale." The whole story is thereby enveloped in secrecy, doubt, and mystery. The mention of the manuscript in the concluding section as the basis for the narrative exerts a distancing effect. Readers are recipients of an oral tradition transmitted to the narrator who mediates his interpretation to us. This may account for the narrator's lack of knowledge about the characters' past; it may also raise doubts about his reliability. Secrets have perhaps been kept from him too.

The intercalation of the manuscript is in keeping with the stylization prevalent throughout *The Scarlet Letter*. For instance, Dimmesdale and Chillingworth are often referred to generically as the "Minister" or the "Physician," although Hester is always given her own name. The triangulated interconnection between them is orchestrated in a consistent pattern of reversals that structure the plot as the initial image of each of the three protagonists undergoes a radical inversion. Hester, first seen in the pillory as the obstinate transgressor, gradually rises in the esteem of both the community and readers as the story progresses. "Disciplined to truth" (167) by the scarlet letter, she shows fortitude in adversity, adamantly refuses to compromise others, and wins admiration for her good deeds. Indeed, she emerges from her tribulations "more saintlike, because the result of martyrdom" (84). Conversely, Dimmesdale and Chillingworth both suffer a sharply negative revision. Chillingworth is intially introduced as "a brilliant acquisition" for the colony because of his familiarity with both traditional medicine and his recently acquired knowledge of Indian herbal remedies. His flagrant misuse of his professional powers for destructive, personally vengeful purposes turns him into a despicable villain. Dimmesdale's metamorphosis is just as dramatic as "the godly pastor" (59) is unmasked as a guilt-ridden sinner. But he is not evil as is Chillingworth. The circumstances and even the location of what happened between him and Hester are among the many facts that remain unknown to readers. Dimmesdale's dual torture by his own conscience and by Chillingworth's manipulation, together with his final public confession, make him pathetic rather than evil. These reversals in their archetypal derivation justify the designation of allegory or parable often applied to *The Scarlet Letter*. Hester is the sinner who becomes saintly; Chillingworth the physician-redeemer turned diabolical, and Dimmesdale the transgressor self-punitive and then repentant.

Such stylization is instrumental in the preponderance of a symbolizing metaphoricity in *The Scarlet Letter*. The surface appearance always carries the potential for a figurative undercurrent, just as the physical symptom has psychological implications. The obvious example of such conflation is

Dimmesdale's reiterated gesture of holding his hand to his heart. This translucence of metaphor in every detail is immediately apparent in the opening section, where the interpenetration of the material and the moral is explicitly voiced. The polar opposition of black flower and rose is continued in the story's structuring tension between darkness and light, gloom and sun, black and red. The dominant somberness of early Puritanism is constantly emphasized, even on a New England holiday: "[T]he gray or sable tinge which undoubtedly characterized the mood and manners of the age" (216); "the sad gray, brown, or black of the English emigrants" (218). The Black Man is the personification of the colonists' superstitious fears. Within this system, the scarlet letter, a sign of a violation, becomes itself a violation of the mandated austerity through its decorativeness, throwing "a lurid gleam along the dark passageway of the interior" (75) of the prison. The defiance represented by the red is a challenge to the authoritarian sway of Puritanism's ascetic sludge hues. The rare appearances of the sun are clearly associated with the break away from Puritanism. At Hester's meeting with Dimmesdale in the forest when she suggests the plan for their escape, as she takes off both the scarlet letter and the formal cap confining her luxuriant hair, "All at once, as with a sudden smile of heaven, forth burst the sunshine, pouring a very flood into the obscure forest, gladdening each green leaf, transmuting the yellow fallen ones to gold" (192–93). But when Hester retrieves the scarlet letter and dons her cap again, "her beauty, the warmth and richness of her womanhood departed, like fading sunshine, and a gray shadow seemed to fall across her" (200).

The portrayal of Dimmesdale's illness is likewise stylized. Because his symptoms are sketched rather than elaborated, their symbolic import is forefronted. The mechanisms of repression, denial, and avoidance underlying conversion disorders are at their most potent in the strict Puritan context of *The Scarlet Letter*. Since ministers played a paramount role in setting moral standards in the colony, Dimmesdale carries a heavy responsibility as a model for his congregation. The social and psychological pressures are therefore particularly stringent on him, and they clash irreconcilably with "the strong animal nature" (128) attributed to him. His heredity thus brings him into conflict with his environment and his conscience. Wedged between his biological instincts and social constraints, Dimmesdale is so utterly bereft of resources that he unconsciously takes to a psychosomatic conversion. His physical decline is at once a substitute and a metaphor for his moral fall. His illness grants him only partially and superficially the primary gain of conversion, namely flight from a situation experienced as intolerable. Its secondary gain derives from not only continued but even heightened admiration from his parishioners and serves, ironically, to aggravate his malaise.

The foil to Dimmesdale's attempt at the formation of a compromise in illness is represented by Hester's staunch acceptance of her guilt and punishment. Her position, too, is biologically determined not merely by her impulsive, passionate temperament but also by the fact that she does not have the choice of concealing her sin when she gives birth to Pearl. Flight into illness is an option hardly available to her. On the other hand, her obligations to her child are a source of strength. In her charitable care of the sick she then extends this altruistic activity, which gives her a sense of self-worth. Her badge of shame comes to be taken for "'Able'"; indeed, she assumes some of Dimmesdale's duties in tending and comforting those in trouble. Because of Pearl, Hester's path is clearer to her. She submits to the Puritan code in being branded by the scarlet letter. But the design of that mark of ignominy is such as to turn it into a decoration—both literally in its beauty and figuratively as a badge of the honor with which Hester bears her lot: "[I]t was so artistically done, and with so much fertility and gorgeous luxuriance of fancy, that it had all the effect of a last and fitting decoration to the apparel which she wore" (60). Hester forms her own kind of compromise, living on the margins of the colony, obedient to its laws, yet at the same time remaining wholly true to her own inner standards of integrity. Her authenticity enables her to face and cope with her situation without denial. She has no secrets from herself, and therefore none of Dimmesdale's necessity for the subterfuges of pretense and illness.

Read from this psychomedical angle, *The Scarlet Letter*'s inter- and intrapersonal dynamics emerge with great clarity. It is a drama of secrets and silences in which the gaze and the gesture take precedence over the utterance. In the tableau at the market place (57–66), the three principal characters eye each other surreptitiously and voicelessly while the throng of spectators staring at Hester in the pillory acts as a chorus. That scene has an eerie echo when Dimmesdale puts himself into the pillory under the cover of darkness. The silences and wary gazes hint at the psychological undergrowth of repression in the avoidance and denial of guilt. The repressed then surfaces in the biological sphere in both Dimmesdale's illness and death and Chillingworth's increasingly sinister decline and disappearance. And the internal conflict of conscience is sharply intensified by the context of Puritanism and the concomitant clash between the moral control mandated within the community and the instinctual naturalness of the surrounding forest. Thus, some hundred and thirty years before Engel formulated the biopsychosocial model, it is well prefigured in *The Scarlet Letter*.

CHAPTER SIX

Nerves: At the Interstices of Physiology and Psychology

Emile Zola, *Thérèse Raquin* (1867)

Everything is itself and at the same time something
else.

—John Banville, *The Untouchable*

"Nerfs" (nerves) is a word that recurs with striking frequency in Zola's early novel *Thérèse Raquin*. Nerves form the mainspring of the actions of the two central characters, the titular Thérèse and Laurent, her lover and subsequently her second husband. Thérèse is at first presented as having the more nervous temperament. Yet, through his association with her, Laurent, too, grows increasingly susceptible to the promptings of his nerves. Acting on the impulsion of their nerves they plot and commit the murder of Thérèse's husband, Camille; although they get away with it, they are locked into a conspiratorial codependency that eventually destroys them.

What was understood by "nerves" at the time of Zola's novel? The meanings of the word had been changing, so that by the mid-nineteenth century it comprised a dualism that is at the heart of *Thérèse Raquin*. Originally, according to the *Oxford English Dictionary*, "nerve" referred literally in the singular to a sinew or tendon and figuratively in the plural to those parts constituting main strength. Secondarily, "nerve" denoted a fiber or bundle of fibers arising from the brain, spinal cord, or other ganglionic organ capable of stimulation by various means, and serving to convey impulses (especially of sensation and motion) between the brain and some other part of the body. Although this secondary sense remains predominantly in the domain of physiology, the somewhat ambiguous word "sensation" suggests a psychological component. This metaphoric potential develops further in the early seventeenth century when "nerve" was used in a nonscientific context in relation to feelings, notably courage or coolness in danger. Such a moral connotation to "nerve" becomes more current in the nineteenth century. For instance, Elizabeth Cady Stanton, rising to make her maiden speech at the Seneca Falls Convention on 19 July 1848, said: "I should feel exceedingly diffident to appear before you at this time, having never before spoken in public, were I not nerved by a sense of right and duty, did I not feel that the time had come for the question of woman's wrongs to be laid before the public."[1] The verbal form "nerved" here carries a positive psychological charge.

The adjective "nervous" underwent a similar transformation. In contrast to the physicalist meanings of the noun, which are still current in medicine, the parallel significations of the adjective have long since become obsolete. The meaning "affecting the sinews" appears only in Middle English, just as "sinewy" and "muscular" went out of use with late Middle English. But from "muscular" it was merely a small step to the figurative "vigorous," "strong," "forcible," "free from weakness, diffuseness," all of which were applied to writings, arguments, and speakers by the first third of the eighteenth century, that is, at the same time as "nerve" expanded to encompass moral attributes. In the late eighteenth and early nineteenth century, with the growing prominence of sensibility concurrent with romanticism, "nervous" described a state of mind conspicuous for the arousal of the nerves. At this point it straddles the physiological and the psychological as well as pleasurable or frightening stimulation.

In their connection to excitability, timidity, and some type of agitation, the new usages pave the way for the application of "nervous" to characterize a disordered state of the nerves. This meaning, increasingly prevalent from the later eighteenth century onward, is common in the medical writings of the third quarter of the nineteenth century at the time of *Thérèse Raquin*. "Nerve" and "nervous" often crop up, as in Zola's novel, in attempts to fathom enigmatic conditions for which no acceptable explanation was available. In part, the difficulty stems from the limitations of medical knowledge and diagnostic capacity at that period. But it resides also in the nature of the phenomena under investigation. In deeming them "psycho-physical,"[2] Daniel Tuke clearly reveals the perplexed bifocalism of his age, the wavering between physiology and psychology that hinges on the dual potential of "nerves."

Tuke represents one fork of the dichotomy in medical opinion in the third quarter of the nineteenth century in his belief in the essential unity of mind and body and the likelihood of their reciprocal influence on each other.[3] Nerves are the medium that bring about nervousness and allied mental states. Unpleasant stimuli enter the body through the senses, traverse its various parts through the nerves, thus causing symptoms.[4] Tuke is unable satisfactorily to elucidate the action of the nerves except by positing the imagination as the conduit for their impact on the mind.

At the opposite end of the medical spectrum to the psychologically oriented Tuke is his American contemporary, George M. Beard.[5] From the outset Beard enthusiastically embraced the physiological line of thought predominant in his day. For him the body takes priority over the mind, and everything hinges on the state of the nerves taken as a corporeal entity. Beard's presentation of neurasthenia is important for its categoric privileging of the physical. In his wholehearted commitment to the physicalist approach Beard is far more in consonance with the trends of his age than Tuke in his pursuit of the imagination. The entire middle ground between body and mind, between somatic lesions or possession by demons as explanations of human behavior remained murky and fraught with confusions. The interdependence of mind and body was observed and intuited (for instance in the many cases of so-called brain fever) though not understood. Nerves were much more amenable to construction in a somatic rather than a psychological sense because this reading was perceived to be underpinned by science, that prime guarantor of credibility.

Medical men's clear preference for physicalist inquiries at mid-century undoubtedly shaped Zola's theoretical exposition of behavior in *Thérèse Raquin*. That science should have made such an impression on him is not surprising in light of the tremendous progress in the understanding of the physiological and pathological functioning of the body taking place at that period. On the other hand, the decisive leap forward in psychology did not occur until Freud's work toward the close of the century.[6] It is therefore wholly in consonance with this cultural context that Zola should opt to envisage nerves as a physiological rather than a psychological entity.

More than most other writers Zola was in touch with the foremost cultural trends of his day. His employment at the major Parisian publishing firm, Hachette, where he became head of publicity, brought him into close contact with the intellectual concerns of the time. The mid- to later nineteenth-century intoxication with science became manifest too in the positivism sponsored by the mathematician Auguste Comte (1798–1853), who maintained that science provides the only valid model of knowledge. The scientific method holds that everything is open to empirical verification in a determined world where phenomena are linked by a strict cause-and-effect chain. The tenets of positivism, notably its complete reliance on logic, its belief in invariable natural laws, and its trust in observation as the basis for proof, turned into a widespread methodology thought to be applicable in every sphere. Zola was subscribing to the ideas of his time when he laid out his views on the action of nerves in the preface to *Thérèse Raquin* as if human behavior could be deduced according to rational rules.

Zola's immediate model, however, was medical: Claude Bernard's *Introduction à l'étude de la médecine expérimentale* (Introduction to the Experimental Study of Medicine), which appeared in 1865, shortly before *Thérèse Raquin*. Bernard was a physician distinguished for his research on the function of the pancreas in digestion and on the relationship of the central and the sympathetic nervous systems. He became the spokesman for the new conception of medicine as a science governed by observation, experimentation, and comparative analysis. For Bernard, medicine's primary locus was the laboratory, where authoritative results could be attained by means of controlled experimentation. The impression made by Bernard on Zola amounted unquestionably to an "influence," for even fifteen years later in his *Le Roman expérimental* (1881; *The Experimental Novel*) Zola still explicitly invokes Bernard. The very title of Zola's work testifies to its derivation from Bernard. Zola argues in *Le Roman expérimental* that the word "novelist" should simply be substituted for the word "doctor" in Bernard's treatise, because the aims and methods of the writer and the medical scientist run parallel. So in *Thérèse Raquin* Zola imagines himself as being in a laboratory conducting an experiment on the physiology of nerves in the two central protagonists. What this self-image disregards is the key presence of the writer's imagination in devising such a pseudo-scientific experiment.

Zola construes the parallelism between doctor and writer in the preface to the second edition to *Thérèse Raquin,* written in 1868, the year after its first publication. Through its open portrayal of sexuality, not to mention murder, the novel aroused furious indignation.[7] Zola was accused of immorality, of being a wretched pervert who took pleasure in displaying human vileness. The preface was added primarily as a defense against the lack of comprehension for his work. Its crux lies in Zola's exposition of his concept of human nature, including the role of nerves in shaping action.

In contrast to his outstanding predecessor in the history of the French novel, Honoré de Balzac—who envisaged himself as a social scientist, the secretary to the nineteenth century in his panoramic chronicle of contemporary society, *La Comédie humaine* (*The Human Comedy*)—Zola chooses a medicalized role for his writerly activity. He declares: "J'ai simplement fait sur deux corps vivants le travail analytique que les chirurgiens font sur les cadavres" (9; I have simply undertaken on two living bodies the analytical work that surgeons perform on cadavers). Zola deliberately alludes to the momentous advances in pathological anatomy to support his use of "la méthode moderne, l'outil d'enquête universelle dont le siècle se sert avec tant de fièvre pour trouer l'avenir" (11–12; the modern method, the universal tool that this century is using so energetically to explore the future). Zola's insistence on the scientific model enables him to rebut the accusation of immorality on the grounds that "[l]e reproche d'immoralité, en matière de science, ne prouve absolument rien" (10; the reproach of immorality proves absolutely nothing in the realm of science). By this shift of focus onto his scientific intention Zola seeks to invalidate the imputations against him. In vain, he laments, has he awaited a voice to proclaim that "'cet écrivain est un simple analyste, qui a pu s'oublier dans la pourriture humaine, mais qui s'y est oublié comme un médecin s'oublie dans un amphithéâtre" (9; this writer is simply an analyst who may have forgotten himself in human rottenness, but who has done so as a doctor forgets himself in a dissecting room). Here again Zola emphasizes the ideal of the pathologist's total detachment, the absence, indeed inappropiateness of either moral judgment or emotional response in the face of the scientific specimen. This is the posture, he maintains, that he has adopted toward his figures. Like or as a scientist, he has engaged in "l'étude d'un cas curieux de physiologie" (8; the study of a curious case in physiology). The words "une étude physiologique" (11; a physiological study) are frequently reiterated in this brief preface together with the term "analyse," often coupled to "scientifique." Zola professes to be showing "pièces d'anatomie nues et vivantes" (12; naked and living pieces of anatomy) "avec la seule curiosité du savant" (10; solely with the researcher's curiosity).

The consequence of such an emphasis on the physiological is an attenuation of the psychological: "J'ai choisi des personnages souverainement dominés par leurs nerfs et leur sang, dépourvus de libre arbitre, entraînés à chaque acte de leur vie par les fatalités de leur chair" (8; I chose people totally dominated by their nerves and their blood, without free will, drawn into each act of their lives by the necessities of their flesh). This supremacy of the physical inevitably entails, as Zola concedes, the eschewal of what he calls the soul: "L'âme est parfaitement absente" (8; The soul is completely absent) so that Thérèse and Laurent are merely "des brutes humaines, rien de plus" (8; human animals, nothing more). Thus Zola affirms his "but scientifique" (8; scientific aim) as being to trace step by step the dictates of instinct that result, as the outcome of a nervous crisis, in "détraquements cérébraux" (8; cerebral derangements). His purpose, described as "l'analyse du mécanisme humain" (9; the analysis of the human mechanism), prompts the reference to the brain (cerebral) rather than to the mind as the site of even hallucinations. Since "l'humanité des modèles disparaissait" (9; the models' human sides disappeared), what would normally be considered their remorse "consiste en un simple désordre organique, en un rébellion du système nerveux tendu à se rompre" (8; consists of a simple organic disorder, a rebellion of the nervous system stretched to breaking point). In underscoring this substitution for "remorse" Zola discloses most clearly his intent to displace psychology in favor of physiology.

In so doing he departs from the tradition known in French as the *roman d'analyse* (analytical novel), which was dedicated to the analysis of subtle intra- and interpersonal feelings. Zola retains the guiding idea of analysis but links it to the medical sciences instead of to humanistic insight. In the rhetorically powerful preface to *Thérèse Raquin* he is in effect espousing a kind of behaviorism based on biological sensations. The impetus to action is corporeal; "nerves," in its original physicalist sense in relation to the body, together with "sang" (blood or instinct) are the determining factors. But although this attempted equation between the writer and the pathologist may be an effective defense against allegations of immorality in *Thérèse Raquin*, it points at once to the novel's intrinsic contradiction: cadavers are devoid of emotion, whereas living beings do have feelings. Even if remorse is categorized as a simple organic disorder, the words "instinct" and, even more so, "nerves" are rife wih psychological connotations. This ambivalence is innate to Zola's novel, and despite his vehement arguments to the contrary, it is precisely for its unintentional illustration of the confluence of the physiological and the psychological that *Thérèse Raquin* is an important text for the literary portrayal of psychosomatic processes. While Zola may have projected an image of himself as an analytic scientist setting up a controlled experiment on the interplay of two temperaments, he is much rather giving an imaginative vision of the mysterious leap from mind to body. The fallaciousness of his analogy between scientist and writer emerges in *Thérèse Raquin* as nerves prove to be an expression less of a physiological than of a psychological crisis.

Zola's attempt to align literature with science is central to naturalism as a literary movement, and nowhere is this aim—and its problematics—more evident than in *Thérèse Raquin*. Zola boldly affirmed that the naturalists "remplacent l'homme métaphysique par l'homme physiologique, et ne le séparent plus du milieu qui le détermine"[8] (replace metaphysical beings with physiological beings, and no longer divorce them from the environment that determines them). The strong preponderance of the physical is apparent throughout the theoretical program of naturalism; its underlying perception of human life devolves from a belief system whose crucial factors are heredity, environment, and the pressure of circumstances (*la race*, *le milieu,* and *le moment*). These three elements were thought to combine with the inevitability of a chemical reaction to produce certain courses of action. So naturalism's model is essentially biosocial, and it rejects psychology. This behavioral paradigm implies an absence of choice that has led to the common criticism of the naturalists' view of life as depriving human beings of free will. While such an inference is to some extent legitimate (or would be if the naturalists had adhered rigidly to their program), in practice the characters in naturalistic writing do make certain choices and have a greater psychological complexity than its theory would admit.

For the determinants of action, though intended as exclusively physical in nature, all comprise strains that transcend the purely substantive. Even the most pronouncedly bodily, heredity, encompasses, besides the corporeal, traits of character or mentality seated in the psyche. Zola himself silently conceded the duality of heredity when he drew up the family tree for *Les Rougon-Macquart* (1871–93), his twenty-volume cycle subtitled *The Natural and Social History of a Family under the Second Empire;* each figure on the elaborate tree is endowed with inherited psychological as well as physical tendencies. Similarly, environment is generally interpreted literally, often with an emphasis on the cramped quarters, the foul smells, and the hunger prevalent in the slums of industrialized cities. But these squalid living conditions have a less tangible dimension too, in the fears, antagonisms, and mechanisms of self-protection and self-indulgence that are an instinctive response to such a setting. Finally, the pressure of circumstances may stem as much from internal as from external stimuli: from desires or apprehensions as from social situations of duress. These ambivalences in the naturalistic creed are often overlooked partly because the exponents of the theory themselves repudiated them. However, scrutiny of any major naturalistic work reveals the impossibility of banishing psychology in favor of physiology. The self-defeating aspect of such an endeavor comes to the fore in *Thérèse Raquin,* first in the double meaning of the word "nerves" and ultimately in the novel's metamorphosis from an experiment in naturalism to an exemplar of sheer Gothic horror.

In the first third of the novel Zola's "experiment" works well enough. He shows the events leading up to the murder as the product of the growing conflict between Thérèse's and Laurent's instinctual sexual drives and their social situation. Thérèse is Camille's wife, Laurent his best friend. The insuperable obstacles to the lovers' meetings drive to them the realization that Camille must be removed, preferably permanently. Yet even in writing about the opening third of *Thérèse Raquin* it is hard to avoid such psychologically laden words as desires, frustrations, and wishes. Obviously, all these feelings are present, although Zola consistently translates them into physical terms.

For instance, Thérèse's urges are explained by the clash between her heredity and her current position. She is the daughter of a sea captain who brought her back to France from Algeria at age two after the death of her mother, a beautiful indigenous woman. Her African origins, her mother's exoticism and hot blood, form the basis for Thérèse's latently passionate nature. The detail included about her rosy cheeks on her arrival also indicates her robust health. Her father hands her over to his sister, Mme. Raquin, and never comes back to visit. So in early childhood Thérèse is abandoned by her father and made to feel unwanted. This brutalization is continued by her aunt, who brings her up alongside her own sickly son, Camille. Thérèse has to share a bed and an invalid life style with her feeble cousin, to whom Mme. Raquin marries her so as to turn her into his nurse.

In the account of Thérèse's personal history two fundamental facts are immediately linked: her innate sensuousness and her obligation to repress this side of herself. She is described as having a feline litheness, taut and powerful muscles, a store of energy and passion lying dormant in her quiescent body.[9] Constantly admonished to keep quiet, Thérèse conceals the impulsive ardor of her nature with supreme self-control so as to maintain an appearance of tranquility. Alone, lying at the water's edge, she is compared to an animal basking in the sun, digging her fingers into the earth, her eyes black and dilated, her body tensed up, ready to spring. From the outset the dangerous split enforced onto Thérèse's being is emphasized, and it is done through notation of her physical movements and her conduct. Her tense body, her dilated eyes, her need to finger the earth hint at the disparity between her surface imperturbability and her suppressed vehemence. Zola focalizes Thérèse from an external perspective; though as an omniscient narrator he implies her feelings, he refrains from explicitly exploring them. The years when she was traumatized and deprived of genuine self-expression through repression of her natural sensuality are vividly but obliquely conveyed in her behavior. The physical is a cipher for the psychological. The outcome of Thérèse's heredity, in conjunction with her subjugation in the Raquin household, is a "tempérament" repeatedly designated as "nerveuse."

Laurent's temperament, on the other hand, is "sanguine" (158). His heredity and situation are far simpler than hers. Of peasant stock, he is large, strong, basically lazy, with simple appetites for food, sleep, and sex, that he wants to satisfy with minimum effort. In physique he is the diametric opposite to the frail Camille: big, with square shoulders, thick black hair, red lips, fresh coloring, and a fleshy neck. Thérèse's instant attraction to him is indicated by the shivers that run through her body as she looks at his firm body and powerful muscles. Not a single syllable is exchanged between them; she cannot take her eyes off him for "elle n'avait jamais vu un homme" (39; she had never seen a man). Thérèse's fascination with Laurent is presented as a biological reaction as predictable and inevitable as that between two complementary chemicals.

The intensity of Thérèse's instinctual drive to Laurent comes even more to the fore through comparison with his relative hesitation. He does not immediately find her physically alluring as she does him. For a whole week he calculates the pros and cons of a liaison with her, finally deciding to embark on it because it is to his own advantage. His peasant-like economy is the clinching argument; with Camille's wife he can satisfy his appetites without cost. And he notes how she quivers for a lover. Their encounter is silent and brutal, like a coupling between animals. Both gratify a physical need without any emotional involvement; their intercourse is simply the assuagement of a sexual drive. Inarticulate creatures, they express themselves through their bodies.

This biological dimension of heredity and instinct clashes with the social dimension of environment. Laurent makes such a tremendous impact on Thérèse because he is the incarnation of life such as had hitherto been denied to her. Zola portrays her existence from the time of her incorporation into the Raquin household until the appearance of Laurent as a living death. This idea pervades the opening description of the street where Mme. Raquin's shop is sited. A long, narrow passage, perpetually dark, humid, full of mold, it at once evokes a coffin. The aura of death is pervasive throughout the first chapter, a still life devoid of movement. The shop itself is likened to a lugubrious hole, its façade "comme couverte d'une lèpre et toute couturée de cicatrices" (16; as if covered with leprosy and all disfigured by scars). The entire setting reeks of decomposition and morbidity. The goods on display are so dusty as to have turned a uniform dirty gray as they too are transformed by the enveloping decay. The three figures silhouetted behind the dirty window pane are as rigid as wax dolls; of the younger woman (Thérèse) only the head is discernible, the body remains out of sight as if it had been completely annihilated by this milieu. The brief chapter is a masterpiece of narrative technique as the narrator's gaze captures the scene like a camera lens zooming in from the street. Direct comment is rendered superfluous by the forcefulness of Zola's images. It is the concrete, physical surface that he records, yet, as in *The Scarlet Letter*, it carries an intense metaphoric undercurrent.

Imprisoned in this sinister, stifling space, tethered to Camille, Thérèse, we readily conclude, experiences her existence as though she had been buried alive. She bears the enclosure forced onto her with an apparently phlegmatic placidity that merely veils temporarily her natural lusts. The exposition of the environment is completed by the portrait of the sole entertainment: the grotesque Thursday evening gatherings of Mme. Raquin's friends. The repetition week after week of the same gestures and phrases underscores the dreary stasis in which Thérèse is trapped. Switching briefly to her perspective, Zola allows a glimpse of her thoughts on these supposedly festive occasions: "[E]lle se croyait enfouie au fond d'un caveau, en compagnie de cadavres mécaniques, remuant la tête, agitant les jambes et les bras, lorsqu'on tirait les ficelles" (36; She thought she was buried in some vault together with mechanical corpses who moved their heads, legs, or arms when the puppets' strings were pulled). So the guests, too, instead of bringing jollity, corroborate the death-like eeriness of this household. Thérèse resorts to the pretext of a bad headache to be excused from the card games, deliberately feigning an indisposition as a means of avoidance. This is the first instance of a psychosomatic disorder in the novel.

The addition of Laurent to this scenario is the catalyst for the explosion previously held in check by lack of opportunity. The tension between Thérèse's de facto captivity and her innate sensuality impels her to adultery. Very quickly the sexual outlet becomes an absolute imperative to both her and Laurent. Zola uses parallel physicalist language to explain their need for each other. In Thérèse's case, "tous ses instincts de femme nerveuse éclatèrent avec une violence inouïe; le sang de sa mère, ce sang africain qui brûlait ses veines, se mit à couler, à battre furieusement dans son corps maigre" (51; all her instincts as a nervous woman burst forth with unprecedented vehemence; her mother's blood, that African blood that burned her veins began to rush and to beat furiously through her thin body). Similarly, Laurent acts "avec une obstination d'animal affamé. Une passion de sang avait couvé dans ses muscles; . . . il obéissait à ses instincts, il se laissait conduire par les volontés de son organisme. . . . Il avait besoin de cette femme pour vivre comme on a besoin de boire et de manger" (65; with the tenacity of a famished animal. A passion in his blood had taken root in his muscles; . . . he obeyed his instincts, he let himself be led along by the demands of his organism. . . . He needed this woman in order to live as one needs to drink and to eat). That the impetus to Thérèse's and Laurent's reciprocal sexual enthralment is primarily physical is entirely credible. "Nerves" function physiologically as expressions of sexual appetites. In murdering Camille, the lovers act under the threat of a loss presented as sensual rather than sentient. So Zola succeeds in motivating their conduct as a physiological response without reference to the psychological aspects.

But after the murder the psychological can no longer be kept so rigorously at bay, even though it continues to appear obliquely in physical signs. Life seems to continue as before in the Raquin household except for the disappearance of Camille. Thérèse's and Laurent's version of the boating "accident" is accepted without question as is her "nervous" collapse immediately after the drowning: "[S]e sentant faible et lâche, craignant d'avouer le meurtre dans une crise, [Thérèse] avait pris le parti d'être malade" (91; Feeling weak and cowardly, afraid of confessing the murder in a moment of crisis, [Thérèse] had chosen the sick role). She repeats here the tactic she had already exploited on Thursday evenings of using illness as a means to avoid an unpleasant or threatening situation. Her disorder at this point may be genuine, though more likely feigned for self-protection. But a strand of emotion appears too: lying there, cowered under the sheets, she experiences anxiety as she listens to what is being said. The more robust Laurent "agissait mécaniquement" (92; acted mechanically), motivated by "l'instinct de conservation" (the instinct for self-preservation) and "des satisfactions de brute" (an animal satisfaction) as he thinks of Thérèse upstairs in bed. Physical manifestations still predominate after the murder: tremblings, twitchings, shudderings, sensations of burning, the contraction of Mme. Raquin's throat when she hears the news. But these are transparent indications of distress, readily interpreted by readers as expressions of inner states of mind.

Still, no great change occurs even after Laurent finally identifies the bloated, greenish, decomposing remains of Camille at the morgue. In his reaction to this horrible sight, the physical again stands in for a possible psychological response; he feels "seulement un grand froid intérieur et de légers picotements à fleur de peau" (100; a cold sensation inside and a slight sense of prickling on his skin). Laurent's sanguine peasant disposition is far hardier than Thérèse's nervous temperament. He grows fat and sloppy, with a big soft body that seems to have neither bones nor sinews/nerves and certainly looks incapable of violence or cruelty. The word "nerfs" (111) is here probably meant to be read in its old connotation of sinews because it is allied to "os" (bones), yet it has the potential of its alternative sense. After a year's interval the lovers are again beset by sexual desire. At the instigation of the Thursday guests, they get married.

Ironically, it is after they have reached the comparative safety of matrimony that their troubles surface, dredged up like their victim's remains from the river. On their wedding night they face each other "anxieux, pris d'un malaise subit" (147; anxious, seized by a sudden malaise). They eye each other "sans désir, avec un embarras peureux, souffrant de rester ainsi silencieux et froids" (148; without desire, in fearful embarrassment at their own silence and coldness). Thérèse throws a strange look of repugnance and fright at Laurent, while he himself is overtaken by terror and disgust. The couple is here responding to each other with feelings, not with the purely physical sensations previously attributed to them. Yet throughout the novel Thérèse and Laurent speak through their bodies. They are poly-symptomatic in their nausea, trembling, pallor, shuddering, palpitations, sweating, insomnia, and chattering teeth, all of which could have a physiological or a psychological causality. The ambiguity contained in the idea of "nerves" pervades the whole of *Thérèse Raquin*.

Far into the narrative Zola tries to uphold the assertion that particularly in Laurent the disturbances are physical, although communicated to him as a contagion from Thérèse's nerves:

> Ses remords étaient purement physiques. Son corps, ses nerfs irrités et sa chair tremblante avaient seuls peur du noyé. Sa conscience n'entrait pour rien dans ses terreurs. . . . Il subissait des crises périodiques de nerfs qui revenaient tous les soirs, qui détraquaient ses sens, en lui montrant la face verte et ignoble de sa victime. On eût dit les accès d'une effrayante maladie, d'une sorte d'hystérie du meurtre. Le nom de maladie, d'affection nerveuse était réellement le seul qui convînt aux épouvantes de Laurent. Sa face convulsionnait, ses membres se roidissaient; on voyait que les nerfs se nouaient en lui. Le corps souffrait horriblement, l'âme restait absente. Le misérable n'éprouvait pas un repentir. (160)

> (His remorse was purely physical. Only his body, his irritated nerves, and his trembling flesh were afraid of the drowned man. His conscience played no part in these terrors. . . . He would undergo periodic attacks, attacks of nerves that recurred every evening, that deranged his senses by confronting him with his victim's green, revolting face. They seemed like attacks of a frightening disease, a sort of murder hysteria. The term "disease," nervous affliction, was really the only one appropriate to Laurent's fits of panic. His face became contorted, his limbs stiff, his sinews could be seen to be all knotted. His body suffered horribly, his soul remained absent. The wretched man felt no repentance).

This passage is crucial for the confluence of the two senses of "nerves." The placement of the phrase "nerfs irrités" in a series between "corps" (body) and "chair" (flesh) shows that it is intended as another physiological element. Similarly, toward the end of the quotation, Laurent's knotted "nerfs" are juxtaposed with his convulsed face, his stiffened limbs, the suffering of his body. Yet the naming of "une effrayante maladie" (a frightening illness), "une sorte de hystérie du meurtre" (a sort of murder hysteria), an "affection nerveuse" (a nervous affliction) also at the same time locates Laurent's condition in the psychological realm.[10] The internal contradiction at the heart of *Thérèse Raquin* can be pinpointed here: between Zola's aim of analyzing the characters in a scientific, medical light, as expounded in the preface, and the novel's undeniable deflection in its latter part into an illustration of the searing effects of guilt.

Zola never ceases to privilege the physical symptoms; mostly he simply eschews actually naming feelings such as remorse, guilt, fear, or anxiety. However, ironically, his very claim that Laurent's soul remained absent and that his conscience played no part in the causation of his discomforts raises the possibility of a moral dimension. Zola repeatedly refers to Thérèse and Laurent as "les meurtriers" (the murderers) and to Laurent as "l'assassin" (208). So he does not attenuate the deed itself, but he masks its psychological sequelae by supplanting them into palpable bodily symptoms. It is as if the writer himself, like his characters, were repressing feelings and converting them instead into corporeal signs.

To some degree this image of Thérèse and Laurent is credible because they are so inarticulate that they hardly have the capacity for verbal expression. Right from the opening still life of three figures silhouetted in the shop-window, the silence in the Raquin household is oppressive. Because of Camille's invalidism, Thérèse is constrained to a quiescence foreign to her nature. The Thursday guests, too, talk little, absorbed in their dominoes, only disputing for two or three minutes between games, "puis le silence retombait, morne" (36; then silence set in again, desolate). No wonder that Thérèse, acculturated to this taciturnity, does not speak to Laurent when she first sees him. Even their love making takes place without the exchange of a single word. Only afterwards does Thérèse speak freely to Laurent of her anger at having been forced to lead "leur vie morte" (54; their dead existence) and of her thoughts of running away to be in the fresh air and sunshine. During the happy days of her affair with Laurent, her tongue is loosened; she jokes, mimics the cat, wondering about the stories it could tell if it could speak.

After the murder, Thérèse's and Laurent's silence is one of fear and complicity. They scrupulously avoid the one topic they need to talk about. It is as if they held the quasi-magical belief that their deed could be abolished, or at least removed from their consciousness, if it is not mentioned. Their joint silence is most harrowing on their wedding night as they sit on opposite sides of the fireplace mute and motionless. At best they utter a few monosyllables, inane words about insignificant matters such as the weather. But beneath this façade, the omniscient narrator tells us, "tout leur être s'employait à l'échange silencieux de leurs souvenirs épouvantés" (150; their whole being went into the speechless exchange of their horrified memories). They stop even their vapid talk out of fear that by chance they will name Camille. They both recognize the potential for a crisis because their nerves "se tendaient" (149; were tensed). The word "tensed" suggests a physical state, and the reflexive verbal form makes it an involuntary action, but the emotional charge is evident. By not speaking, they pretend to have forgotten the past, but their avoidance only fosters repression. Although they refuse to hear their "voix intérieure" (205; inner voice), pre-sumably the voice of their guilty conscience, they cannot control the man-ifestations of their bodies: "le corps s'était révolté, . . . ils tendaient leurs nerfs, ils se roidissaient sans parvenir à se délivrer" (205; their bodies had rebelled, . . . they tensed their nerves, they stiffened, but without succeed-ing in freeing themselves). Their habit of converting repressed emotions into physiological reactions is cogently motivated as an attempted means of avoidance.

Language is replaced in *Thérèse Raquin* by the gaze. Thérèse's eyes are glued to Laurent when he first appears, and from then on, both before and after the murder they communicate by looks and gestures, although even-tually they reach a point where they do not dare to look at each other. The gaze takes on a sinister role when Mme. Raquin becomes paralyzed and bereft of speech by a stroke. She then actually *is* the wax figure she had seemed to be in the initial tableau. After she learns the facts about her son's death when Thérèse and Laurent openly quarrel about the murder in her presence, her watching, accusatory gaze becomes a central element of the novel's horror. Another beholding eye, that of the cat, strikes Laurent as so menacing that he hurls it out of the window up against a wall where its head shatters. The novel ends, as it had begun, on Mme. Raquin's immo-bile figure as she contemplates Thérèse's and Laurent's corpses. This final picture brings *Thérèse Raquin* to a fitting closure in the ultimate triumph of the silent gaze. This concluding tableau is also a reprise, with variations, of the opening one: now Thérèse is really dead instead of only looking so; Laurent has replaced Camille; and Madame Raquin's speechless watchful-ness has become a pathological aphonia.

The silences and the replacement of speech by gaze are credible because Thérèse and Laurent are in many ways simple creatures, neither self-aware nor given to reflection, though not the mere animals ("bêtes") in human form that Zola posits for his naturalistic experiment. What changes them after the murder is their reciprocal dependency, their per-nicious bonding through a secret that they endeavor to conceal not only from others but from their own consciousness too. That secret becomes pathogenic in a kind of bondage. Even as Zola professes to be portraying bodies with nerves, he is actually uncovering psychological mechanisms in physical forms. As the two drift into psychotic hallucinations, their apprehension of reality is undermined and distorted by their fixation on the gruesome memory of the drowned Camille. Interestingly, in characters who are nonverbal, it is the visual impact that haunts them. They are so obsessed with the greenish, rotting corpse of their victim that they sense his damp presence lying between them in bed. When Thérèse becomes pregnant, she has a vague fear of delivering a drowned creature. She thinks she can feel in her innards the coldness of a soft, decomposing corpse. She has a miscarriage as a result of Laurent's violent blow to her abdomen. Their earlier sexual magnetism now turns into a complex amalgam of repulsion and a kind of negative fixation. Each wants to part from the other in order to escape from their threatening secret, yet it is precisely that secret that yokes them as partners in crime. The long duration of the stress under which they labor without prospect of an escape or end drives them to the breaking point. Their simultaneous plans to murder each other culminate in a melodramatic double suicide. As they drop dead on the floor, Thérèse's mouth lands on the scar of the wound Camille's teeth had inflicted on Laurent's neck, that powerful neck that had so fascinated her at first sight. Their joint death is a version or a perversion of the nineteenth-century *Liebestod,* the climax to Wagner's *Tristan and Isolde,* first performed just two years before *Thérèse Raquin.*

The wound on Laurent's neck functions as the visible, indelible reminder of culpability. Inscribed on his body, it will not heal, standing out red and ugly, and repeatedly activating Thérèse's revulsion. It also carries a mythical undercurrent in its reference to the mark of the biblical Cain. Thus the site of Thérèse's primary attraction to Laurent is metamorphosed into the symbol of her aversion and their mutual guilt. The wound is an outstanding example of Zola's practice of translating the psychological into the physical.

In portraying his characters from this behavioristic perspective, Zola is as a writer replicating exactly what they are doing: turning the psychological into the physical. If their bodily self-expressions are indications of sexual arousal before the murder, after it they are clearly idioms of distress. While Thérèse and Laurent want to deny their guilt, the image of the drowned Camille becomes a fixed idea that they cannot excise. Even as they avoid acknowledging the nature of their deed, the memory returns insistently as a profoundly destructive force. They hear their own sobs as their victim's mocking laughter. Their expectation of happiness and sexual fulfillment once Camille is out of the way turns into a nightmare in which they torture themselves as much as each other. Their joint suicide, a desperate means of escape, is at the same time a form of self-punishment for a guilt they cannot avow but that dogs them nonetheless.

So the physical disturbances that Thérèse and Laurent exhibit in the novel's latter half can easily be identified as veiled evidence of distress, externalizations of the inner feelings they are repudiating. All the tremblings and such are displaced feelings, projections into the body of terrors that the psyche is unable to face. As such they are classical conversion phenomena, functioning as substitutes for emotions that the protagonists dare not concede, let alone pronounce. In the manner characteristic of psychosomatic disorders, the body becomes the carrier of an overwhelming pain too ghastly to utter.

In its consistent transliteration of the psychological into the physiological *Thérèse Raquin* affords a remarkable example of conversion disorder. The ambiguity of the key word "nerves" allows for the conflation of the physical and the mental. Zola's beliefs lead to the supplanting of inner feelings by outward symptoms, thereby reproducing typical psychosomatic processes. Flesh and blood, sinews and tendons are the pathways for the discharge of desires, anxieties, and fears.

Yet this claim itself suggests the self-defeating aspect of Zola's methodology, which in this respect too parallels the course of psychosomatic illness. For the underlying psychological core of both Zola's characters and of psychosomatic disorders cannot ultimately be banished. Nerves stand not only for anatomical parts but also for mental responses to a variety of generally frightening situations. Readers of *Thérèse Raquin* have no difficulty in carrying out a reverse translation to that performed by Zola; they automatically recognize in Thérèse's and Laurent's tremblings and the like the feelings for which they stand: sexual excitement at the beginning, and then fear, anxiety, rising to a crescendo of unbearable terror by the end. In this regard *Thérèse Raquin* departs from the customary model of works that portray psychosomatic disorders. Normally readers (like therapists) are required to undertake a detective search for the covert sources of the disturbance. In this case readers know its origins in the murder. Although Zola rejects the notion of conscience in his claim that the soul is absent, its forceful presence is evident to readers who envisage nerves in the psychological connotation as much as in the physiological sense that Zola places in the foreground. Thus readers simultaneously engage with the text and disengage from the narrator in perceiving the psychological within the physiological.

So, as the Irish writer John Banville very aptly phrased it in his novel *The Untouchable* (1997), "*[E]verything is itself and at the same time something else*" (45). This formula could in fact be the motto for all psychosomatic disorders: the physical symptoms are unquestionably real to the sufferer but also denote an ulterior problem on the psychological level. Zola, in his purported role as anatomist, strives in *Thérèse Raquin* to abolish that psychological dimension. He consistently forefronts the biological and social etiology of Thérèse's and Laurent's disorders by emphasizing their lower, animalistic sides. So long as the drive is primarily sexual, this conception remains plausible enough. However, in the latter part of the novel, the characters' "soul" is not absent: the sources of their morbidity are quite evident. Their nerves are not merely conditioned physiological reactions but sentient psychological responses. Even though their inner distress is projected into bodily manifestations, readers recognize them as "*at the same time something else.*" Nerves are here at once physiological and psychological. If initially they form the primary impulse to eros, ultimately they also determine the impetus to thanatos.

CHAPTER SEVEN

"A Sick Spot on the Body of the Family"

Thomas Mann, *Buddenbrooks* (1901)

> All happy families are alike, each unhappy family is
> unhappy in its own way.
>
> —Tolstoy, *Anna Karenina*

"**D**u bist ein Auswuchs, eine ungesunde Stelle am Körper unserer Familie!"[1] (You are a sore, a sick spot on the body of our family), Thomas shouts at his profligate younger brother in an angry confrontation. The German word "Auswuchs" has a sinister ring, suggesting something ugly, a growth that should not be there, possibly even a malignancy. Christian is certainly the most glaringly aberrant among the Buddenbrooks, but he is by no means the only sick spot in the family. With its abundance of disease and illness *Buddenbrooks* opens up the slippery borderlands where somatic and psychosomatic disorders intersect. It also affords the ideal opportunity to apply the biopsychosocial model because of its richly vivid evocation of the social context and its demonstration of the impact that environment has on all its main characters.

Buddenbrooks is the quintessential family saga. Spanning the forty years between 1835 and 1875, it follows the lives of four generations of Buddenbrooks. The personal happenings—the marriages, births, deaths, and divorces—are embedded in the political, economic, and social transformation of Germany during the mid-nineteenth century. The protagonists discuss and are affected by the 1848 revolution, the Schleswig-Holstein War of 1866, the extension of the German Customs Union, the introduction of gas street lighting, growing industrialization, the founding of the North German Confederation in 1867, the Austro-Prussian War of 1870, the expansion of the railroad network, the eclipse of the old-style patricians, and the concomitant empowerment of a new capitalist bourgeoisie.[2] These events form not merely the backdrop to the unfolding of the plot; they impinge directly on the family. In 1848, for example, the maid bursts into the dining room to stage her own disruptive revolt; in 1870 Prussian officers are billeted in the Buddenbrook residences. Such episodes function both as markers of the passage of historical time, reminding readers of the long duration of the novel's action, and as demonstrations of the effect of political events on private lives.

Through this lengthy time span Mann is able to show the cumulative changes that overtake the Buddenbrooks in the course of four generations as well as the etiology of their sicknesses. The work's original title, *Verfall* (Decline), which was expanded in the final subtitle to *Verfall einer Familie* (Decline of a Family) announces its central theme. The action begins symbolically, with the festivities to celebrate the Buddenbrooks' move into a splendid house, acquired from a family whose fortunes had waned. The same fate eventually overtakes the Buddenbrooks themselves, so that they have to sell the house to the up-and-coming Hagenströms. Rise and decline are thus represented as cyclical recurrences. After a glorious phase of dominance in the city's business and social circles, the Buddenbrooks increasingly lose their financial acumen, indeed, their interest, in their once preeminent firm. In the third generation already and even more markedly in the fourth, devotion to aesthetic pursuits overrides the earlier commitment to commerce. And as their self-confidence wanes and their tendency to introversion grows, various forms of ill health proliferate. Mind and body are as intimately connected throughout *Buddenbrooks* as are individuals and their environment.

The milieu is the decisive "intervening variable"[3] in this novel.[4] For this reason the insistent depiction of its manifestations and effects is of such cardinal importance. More than just a physical place, it embraces a whole way of living and thinking that fundamentally shapes the characters' beliefs, responses, attitudes, and conduct. Though never actually named in the text, the city is clearly identifiable from its streets and landmarks as Lübeck, Mann's hometown, one of the five independent city-states that constituted the Hanseatic League. An austere North German Protestant work ethic predominates in the pervasive pressure to financial success; precise calculations of the Buddenbrook firm's assets and cash worth punctuate the narrative. This is a decidedly conservative but not static society. Two factors in the Buddenbrooks' decline are Thomas's adherence to his forefathers' business practices, and his catastrophic failure when he ventures into the kind of risk taking that the Hagenströms master so well.

Thomas clings with such tenacity to the principles inculcated into him out of a determination to maintain the ethos traditional to his family and his culture. The stamp of capitalism is imprinted in the emphasis on money, the sumptuousness of the meals, the luxuriousness of the houses and their furnishings as well as their inhabitants' clothing and habits. The social layering is indicated too by the workers' Low German dialect speech as against the owners' interspersal of French phrases into their conversations.[5] The reiterated references to the "first families" with their round of weekly and annual rituals are constant reminders of the hierarchical nature of this social order. But some at least of the snobbery is grounded in a system of genuine values. While ambition and prominence (for instance, in the city's government) are important, so is strict observance of what is considered as propriety and decorum. For the customary social institutions are more than mere expressions of etiquette; they carry a deeper meaning in denoting assent to the consensually approved lifestyle. However, propriety and decorum may degenerate into the imperative just to keep up appearances ("die Dehors wahren"). In part such a practice is obviously a form of hypocrisy that subverts the very essence of the authenticity it is supposed to support; yet, from another angle, it can also be interpreted as a tribute to the force of the ethos that continues to exert its influence. And a cardinal component of keeping up appearances is a staunch stoicism, a front of silent endurance whatever the psychological cost to the individual.

This is the context in which Christian is branded as "a sick spot on the body of our family," because he blatantly transgresses all the codes of conduct to which, as a Buddenbrook, he is expected to conform. The immediate provocation for Thomas's condemnation is Christian's assertion at the Gentlemen's Club that all businessmen are swindlers. This amounts to a direct affront, a betrayal, indeed an indictment of the standards of integrity pivotal to Thomas himself and to the family concept of honor. Christian's facetious derision marks him as a traitor and confirms his status as an outsider to the family and to the accepted social norms.

Christian's outburst is the culmination of his refractory behavior ever since childhood. He does not take school seriously, absorbed instead in his passion for the theater and in showing off his gift for mimicry. In his adolescence he spends his pocket money on a bouquet for an actress that he presents at the stage door, an audacious act that mobilizes the family's horrified disapproval as a sign of his frivolous temperament and unholy inclinations. Not attracted to commerce, he considers studying law or medicine, but never settles into any profession. His eight years in an apprenticeship in a London firm are followed by a protracted stay in South America. These travels are motivated less by any desire to acquire skills than by the urge to distance himself from the sphere of the family. Soon after his return to Germany he is off to Hamburg. Incapable of sustained effort, he lasts no more than a short time in any workplace. When Thomas tries to employ him for English correspondence, he arrives late, smokes, reads the newspaper, and disappears at the lunch break. He leads the "chaotic life" often found in somatizers.[6] His flightiness and disdain of business strike the family as so reprehensible as to be scandalous.

Christian tries to escape the burden of his obligations as a Buddenbrook by literal and metaphorical flight. His avoidance of his hometown is one means to elude his family's censure. Another is the flight into illness; Christian exhibits an unending stream of symptoms in several parts of his body. His complaints fit perfectly *DSM-IV*'s diagnostic criteria for conversion disorder: "deficits affecting voluntary motor or sensory function that suggest a neurological or medical condition"; they are ills hard to diagnose that cannot be explained by any of the doctors Christian consults; they are not feigned; they produce significant distress and impairment; and "psychological factors are judged to be associated with them."[7]

Christian acquires experience of the sick role early in life. His very first appearance in the opening chapter of *Buddenbrooks* shows him in the throes of an acute bout of indigestion. Stomach pains and nausea force the child to leave the overabundant dinner to celebrate the family's move into their new house. The governess accompanies him, and soon his mother comes to see what is the matter, as does the family physician, a guest at the feast. From this episode Christian learns one of the lessons that will determine his adult behavior: the effectiveness of illness as an attention-attracting device. This is the only time in his childhood that Christian is in the limelight without competition from his siblings. In this incident he also already reveals his proclivity to exaggeration as he loudly vows that he will never ever eat again. This histrionic streak in his personality is a trait frequently associated with somatization disorder,[8] and one that will foster his inclination to display his ailments within his family in spectacular manifestations at once comic and grotesque.

The little ordinary childhood indisposition sets the pattern for Christian's subsequent series of psychosomatic disorders. As Alexander points out, precursory transitory symptoms at an early age are likely to develop during times of emotional stress and to recur whenever new conflict situations arise.[9] So in late adolescence, the period when the formation of personal identity is to be accomplished, Christian enacts choking on a peach stone stuck in his throat: "'Denkt euch, wenn ich aus Versehen . . . diesen grossen Kern verschluckte, und wenn er mir im Halse steckte . . . und ich nicht Luft bekommen könnte . . . und ich spränge auf und würgte grässlich, und ihr alle spränget auch auf. . . .' Und plötzlich fügte er ein kurzes, stöhnendes 'Oh' hinzu, das voll ist von Entsetzen, richtet sich unruhig auf seinem Stuhle empor und wendet sich seitwärts, als wollte er fliehen" (56; "Just think if by mistake I . . . were to swallow this big stone, and if it were to stick in my throat . . . and I couldn't get air . . . and I were to jump up and choke horribly, and you would all jump up too. . . ." And suddenly he added a short moaning "Oh," full of terror, rises anxiously in his chair, and turns as though he wanted to flee.) Christian's projection, prompted by his hyperactive imagination and his theatrical talent, is so compelling that he actually convinces himself of the possibility of such an accident and experiences vehement fear. He literally talks himself into the crisis. The wholly conjectural nature of this scenario is made explicit by the use of rather unusual, weighty subjunctive forms in German ("spränge," "würgte"), and its drama is heightened by the abrupt switch to the present tense as he "rises" from his chair. Christian evokes the hypothetical situation with such vividness as to scare his mother and governess. This scene is in several respects a repetition of the childhood indigestion: it occurs at the family dinner table; it concerns harm done by the ingestion of food; it includes again a vow never to eat again, this time albeit limited to peaches; and, above all, it alarms those close to him. No longer a child, Christian becomes even more aware of the manipulative potential of illness as a means to gain attention and possibly to arouse his family's sympathy.

Christian's descent into illness is in counterpoint to his brother's rise to eminence following his splendid match with the wealthy Gerda Arnold-sen. Not coincidentally, this is the time when Christian develops, in addition to the paralysis of his swallowing muscles, an indeterminate, plaguing pain in his left side that Dr. Grabow is totally at a loss how to treat. Throughout the rest of his life, Christian harps on the description of the sensation: "'Es ist kein Schmerz . . . so kann man es nicht nennen', erklärte er mühsam, indem er mit der Hand an dem Beine auf und nieder fuhr, seine grosse Nase krauste und die Augen wandern liess. 'Es ist eine Qual, eine fortwährende, leise, beunruhigende Qual im ganzen Bein . . . und an der linken Seite, an der Seite, wo das Herz sitzt. . . . Sonderbar ... ich finde es sonderbar!'" (246; "It isn't exactly a pain, I couldn't call it that," he explained laboriously, running his hand up and down the leg, wrinkling his big nose and letting his eyes roam. "It's a torture, a continuous, low-grade, disturbing torture in the whole leg . . . and on the left side, the side where the heart resides. . . . Strange . . . I find it strange!"). This lament recurs in ever more operatic tirades after the birth of a son to Thomas and his election to the city Senate. His brother's success and the respect he wins in the city are undoubtedly sources of stress to Christian. However much he tries to detach and remove himself physically from his native environment, he cannot really do so because of the name he bears. In contrast to Thomas's increasing prestige, Christian is the good-for-nothing, whose only idiom for the expression of his distress is illness.

As he ages prematurely and continues to dwell compulsively on his ailments, Christian becomes a figure of fun and an object of contempt. His adoption of the sick role fails to achieve its purpose in the long run. Paralleling his by now boring recital of his afflictions is the narrator's mockery of him: "Die Sache war die, dass Christian jetzt mehr als jemals Herr seiner Zeit war, denn wegen schwankender Gesundheit hatte er sich genötigt gesehen, auch seine letzte kaufmännische Tätigkeit, die Champagner- und Kognakagentur fahrenzulassen" (564; The fact was that Christian was now more than ever master of his time, for, owing to his precarious health, he had been forced to give up his last business activity as an agent for champagne and cognac.) The dry tone, as of a factual report, is undermined by the irony in the use of the passive tense which allows Christian to appear a victim of his ill health while implying just the opposite.

Christian's case is quite transparent. His multiple complaints, which come to dominate his life, are the flags of and metaphors for his dis-ease in the Buddenbrook family. His social situation combines with his personality to define his behavior. His discomfort stems in part at least from his awkward place in the Buddenbrooks's third and central generation: as the second son and the third child, he lives the shadow of his older siblings, Tom and Tony (Antonie). From his childhood onward, he is always paired with Tom, who is destined, as the eldest, to become head of the family and the firm, while Christian is, by birth sequence, consigned to a lesser position. The unfavorable comparison with the serious-minded Tom, who enters the business at the age of sixteen, immediately sets up a yardstick by which Christian is bound to be seen as falling short. At the birth of their younger sister, for instance, Thomas is given an elegant leather briefcase, whereas Christian receives a puppet theater. As an adult, in one of his confrontations with Tom, Christian reproaches his brother: "'Du bist unseren Eltern immer der bessere Sohn gewesen'" (491; "You were always the better son to our parents"). Evidently, from an early age on, Christian suffers from the hurt occasioned by his relegation to a secondary position in the family, although only much later is he able to articulate his resentment. It is precisely his long repression of his animosity toward his brother and the family ethos Tom represents that is fertile ground for his proclivity to somatize.

Illness therefore becomes a channel for Christian to assert an identity of his own, even if it has to be defined oppositionally and negatively. While his elder sister merely deems him a little peculiar, Tom is relentlessly judgmental of Christian's lack of seriousness and his shamelessness. His Bohemian habits and friends, his readiness to act the clown, to regale any willing listeners with gross tall tales are the stark antithesis to the dour self-control prized by the Buddenbrooks. Christian is an embarrassment to the family, not least in his constant production of his symptoms. The more rejection he suffers, the more he revels, as if in revenge, in challenging the prescribed codes of conduct. In contrast to Tom's socially and financially brilliant match, Christian has a lengthy relationship (and an illegitimate child) with a woman of dubious standing.

This disparity between Tom's and Christian's respective marriages not only epitomizes the discrepancy between their social acceptability but also points to the psychological springs of Christian's actions. For his marriage, like many of his other aberrant actions, is a demonstrative defiance of his family, almost as if he were driven by a perversely destructive and self-destructive impetus. He tries to neutralize the feelings he fears and represses by contrary behavior that puts him beyond the pale, and thus beyond comparison too. For his primary dread is comparison with his brother, since it would inevitably show him up as a ridiculous failure. By deliberately pursuing a course that leads his family and his community to see him as a disgrace, he masks his anxiety about his deep-seated sense of his own inadequacy. This is the secret motivation for his rejection of the Buddenbrook expectations. He will not compete so as not to face confirmation of his suspicion that he is somehow wanting. Unable to meet conventions, he compensates by flagrantly flaunting them.

Christian's secret is never voiced, nor is he portrayed as admitting it to himself. This is partly an outcome of the narrational disposition that withholds from Christian the indirect discourse accorded to Thomas and Tony. So while readers have ready access to their thoughts at crucial points in their lives, Christian is always seen from the outside as perceived by others. He is envisaged from different perspectives, through the eyes of various members of his family as well as those of the narrator. Thus readers' knowledge of him is circumscribed by the actions we see and the words he utters. He is certainly not inarticulate, as are Thérèse and Laurent in *Thérèse Raquin*; he has quite the opposite tendency to hold forth interminably, but he speaks of his symptoms, not his feelings. His self-awareness is channeled to a pathological extent into observation of his physical state, while his innermost reflections remain veiled. Tom finds it abhorrent that Christian "sein Innerstes nach aussen kehrt" (223; turns his intimate side outward), yet Christian does so only by discharging his distress via his body. Although he is vociferous in his minute elaboration of his physical symptoms, the implicit psychological distress at the root of his behavior is not voiced. On the other hand, he is by no means lacking in psychological insight. His occasional comments, such as his jealousy of Thomas for having been the preferred son, betray a glimpse of his hurt ego, and later in life his anger will irrupt into a violent outburst against Thomas.

But Christian never realizes the connection between his chronic bodily complaints and his persistent dissatisfaction with his place in his family and his social context. Without the entry into his mind afforded by indirect discourse it is impossible to know how much he really knows about himself. Perhaps he is to all appearances shameless in the conduct of his life as a disguise for the unavowed shame he does feel. His rebellion against the ethos in which he was raised is rooted in a combination of his unwillingness and his incapacity to meet its demands. Christian dimly intuits this shortcoming and cannot deal with his guilt other than by conversion into illness, which provides the secondary gain of exemption from work and eventually from family expectations as he is written off as "a sick spot." When he becomes the butt of the narrator's irony too, the universal disapproval is complete.

Christian has generally been cast as a subsidiary character in *Buddenbrooks*; his centrality to the novel has not been fully recognized. Indeed, he has been treated by critics in much the same way as by his family. At first, attention focused on the scandal created when Mann's uncle claimed that he was the model for Christian and threatened action for libel.[10] Later, he was described as "Mann's first essay in caricaturing the spirit which has broken away from the business of seriously living and willing."[11] A subtler understanding emerges from the observation that "Christian's broad family head and large nose make him too homely for stardom. He specializes in character roles; he is particularly adept at Anglo-American forms of comedy."[12] But the significance of his "chronic but fluctuating"[13] psychosomatic disorders as emblematic of the novel's overarching theme of decline has never been adequately explored.

Christian is far from being the only "sick spot on the body of our family" or in fact the only one given to putting on a performance. Thomas, who aspires to be the model Buddenbrook, proves even more complex than Christian and ultimately as severely debilitated. It is an appropriate irony that Christian alone has the capacity to see through Thomas in a recognition of the likeness of the apparently other.

In the "murderous . . . sibling rivalry"[14] between Thomas and Christian, the elder brother is the self-righteous incarnation of the Buddenbrook ideal. Engrossed in business, ever mindful of the firm's need for capital, proper, well-groomed, married to a beautiful heiress, owner of a palatial new house, elected to the city senate, father of a son, highly respected in the community: Thomas appears to be the very incarnation of success. Yet, from his youth on, signs of stress in his life are evident, for instance in his enduring addiction to the strong Russian cigarettes he smokes incessantly, inhaling deeply. This compulsive habit may be an attempt to soothe the nervousness that dogs him. His nervousness is a reiterated motif throughout the novel, hinting, like his need to smoke, at hidden tensions. As the guardian of the Buddenbrook heritage, Thomas carries the burden of a responsibility that weighs heavily on him.

In contrast to Christian, Thomas maintains a façade that is in every respect impeccable. But it is a façade, and gradually it comes to function as a mask. The elegance of his appearance, described in his youth already as conspicuous, degenerates into a consuming passion. The house he builds has an exceptionally large dressing-room, where he spends a disproportionate amount of time on his grooming, changing shirts several times a day. While Thomas angrily deprecates Christian's disgusting self-observation, it becomes apparent that he himself is no less prone to this failing in his dandyism.

In the long run, the dichotomization of Thomas and Christian throughout *Buddenbrooks* turns out to be a smoke screen. The resemblance between them is greater than first meets the eye, and it is perhaps the recognition on both sides of that dark kinship that sharpens the conflict. For Thomas, like Christian, is putting on an act. Christian's is the more obvious and the more spontaneous; his long-standing attraction to the theater is a resonance of his own theatricality. Thomas's ploys are considerably more surreptitious and devious. To act out the Buddenbrook ethos is the central mission of his life, and he has to persist in this course long after he has lost faith in his ability to do so. His secret is thus similar to Christian's, although it is more bitter because he has tried and failed, whereas Christian has never tried. The business languishes under Thomas's direction, his wife takes refuge in music from a marriage lacking intimacy, his son proves a terrible disappointment.

Hollowed out and exhausted by the constant efforts required to sustain the façade, Thomas comes merely to impersonate the Buddenbrook ideology instead of being its foremost carrier. His "self-production is self-protection"[15] as he concentrates on his largely successful endeavor to keep his image intact. He is obsessive-compulsive in pursuit of a single aim: to maintain outer appearances. The symbol for the tension between his immaculate surface and his inner despondency is the mask. Thomas is adept at donning it, together with fresh clothes, as a prop of his public persona, like an actor who steps onto the stage in an artfully perfected costume. But once the performance is over, he sags:

> Die Muskeln des Mundes und der Wangen, sonst diszipliniert und zum Gehorsam gezwungen, im Dienste einer

unaufhörlichen Willensanstrengung, spannten sich ab, erschlafften; wie eine Maske fiel die längst nur noch künstlich festgehaltene Miene der Wachheit, Umsicht, Liebenswürdigkeit und Energie von diesem Gesichte ab, um es in den Zustand einer gequälten Müdigkeit zurückzulassen; . . . ohne Mut zu dem Versuche, auch sich selbst noch zu täuschen, vermochte er von allen Gedanken, die schwer, wirr und ruhelos seinen Kopf erfüllten, nur den einen, verzweifelten festzuhalten, dass Thomas Buddenbrook mit zweiundvierzig Jahren ein ermatteter Mann war. (369)

(The muscles of his mouth and cheeks, usually well controlled and forced to obedience in the service of the incessant exercise of his will-power, relaxed and grew slack; like a mask, the expression of alertness, attention, geniality, and energy, long upheld only as an artifice, dropped away to leave his face in a state of tortured fatigue; . . . without the courage for the attempt at further self-deception, of all the thoughts that filled his head in somber, swirling confusion, he could hold on to just the one desperate realization, that Thomas Buddenbrook at age forty-two was a worn-out man.)

The passage is interesting from several points of view. It shows Thomas, too, speaking through his body, as he yields to his real self when out of the public eye. It is also important for granting readers insight into his mind and his hidden tragedy. Despite the differences between them, the two brothers have an ulterior affinity. Far from being his opposite, Christian is a complementary, cautionary figure to Thomas, a parodistic other who lets himself go, whereas Thomas imposes stringent self-discipline on himself. Seen in this light, Thomas's vehement attacks on Christian are expressions not only of outrage but also of fear—fear of the covert likeness between them. They share the same secret in their incapacity to live up to the Buddenbrook ideal. But they devise divergent ways of dealing with it: Christian flamboyantly externalizing his nonconformity in his Bohemianism and his illnesses, while Thomas does his utmost to preserve a semblance of conformity. Christian grows thinner, Thomas stouter. But Thomas's strength wanes; a vacation at the seaside, ordered by his doctor to combat his nervousness, is of no avail. When he is suddenly felled by a stroke following a botched tooth extraction, his death is the physical consummation of a process of psychological dissolution long under way. Repression takes a fatal toll on Thomas. Christian, who has diverted his distress outward into his bodily ailments, survives him, albeit in the insane asylum to which his wife has committed him.

The real survivor in this family is Tony. Significantly, she is the only persona present in both the novel's opening and closing chapters. Tony is tragicomic in her loyalty to "the family and the firm," a phrase constantly on her lips as her guiding motto. Her immense pride in being a Buddenbrook leads her to look down on "upstarts" like the Hagenströms and to expect homage from them for her lofty social status. Although she is very much shaped by the dominant ethos, she fails wretchedly in her efforts to live up to it and to bring honor to the family. Like Thomas, she sacrifices her first and only true love in order to make a socially approved match. But both her marriages end in divorce, and her disgrace is compounded by her son-in-law's imprisonment for fraud. On the door of the small apartment she inhabits at the end with her daughter and granddaughter, she styles herself "Widow Buddenbrook." This curious designation is in a sense fitting, for she is the widow of the Buddenbrooks' glory.

Yet even Tony, the healthiest of the third Buddenbrook generation, has a recurrent psychosomatic disorder. She is subject to attacks of a nervous weakness of her stomach that initially surfaces during her first marriage to a man for whom she feels a deep revulsion. That feeling translates into digestive disturbances, a metaphoric physical counterpart to her aversion to her husband. In a manner typical of somatoform disorders, her affliction fluctuates with the vicissitudes of her life, disappearing when she is hopeful and returning in phases of unhappiness. During her second marriage in Munich, where the strangeness (to her) of the food symbolizes her rejection of the entire culture, her body is the register of her sense of alienation in a foreign milieu whose easygoing ethos is bewildering to her. After her second divorce, as her life sinks into dreariness, her stomach becomes more troublesome; when the Hagenströms are lauded as the cream of society, she has violent cramps. Later she develops another nervous tic: a dry clearing of her throat. Seemingly always buoyant, Tony nonetheless has griefs that she vents through her body.

With Hanno, the only fourth-generation male Buddenbrook, the family becomes extinct. From his birth onward Hanno is presented in great detail and through his own thoughts as well as through the eyes of others. Destined to succeed his father, Thomas, in the business, he is early taken to the firm's warehouses and the wharfs to be taught the names of the grain-carrying ships. But Hanno is much more potently drawn to his mother's music-making, to which he listens with rapt attention, than to business affairs, of which he absorbs nothing. A hypersensitive, fragile child, Hanno suffers from night terrors and bad teeth and hates school, where he does badly.

Hanno's death from typhoid fever is one of the most memorable chapters in this long novel. In sharp contrast to the extensive human details at his grandmother's and his father's deathbeds, Hanno's passing is brief and wholly impersonal in manner. The three-page chapter opens with: "Mit dem Typhus ist es folgendermassen bestellt" (645; This is the course of typhus). The unfolding of the disease is recorded with a factuality and clinical detachment such as might be found in a medical textbook. The sequential stages of the fever, its normative progression, the customary supportive interventions, and the prognosis are catalogued with the objectivity characteristic of a medical textbook. Not even the patient's name is given; only in the novel's final chapter, whose action takes place some six months later, do we learn, almost incidentally, that the victim was Hanno.

Hanno's death could be taken as an unfortunate coincidence, were it not for the framework of the novel's theme of inexorable decline. Enteric fevers were epidemic in Europe at the time of the action of *Buddenbrooks;* several members of the British royal family, including Queen Victoria's husband, succumbed to typhoid. A plausible source of Hanno's infection is skillfully intercalated when the young Hagenströms, in rough and rather threatening horseplay, shove Hanno's head under the water in the pond where they are bathing. Hanno probably swallowed some contaminated water. But this is likely to be overlooked by readers who see the incident more as a symbolic illustration of the Hagenströms' robustness and ruthlessness than as the possible cause of Hanno's illness.

The common interpretation of Hanno's fatal fever is as a willed suicide. He dies of an opportunistic infection because he has lost the will to live, certainly to live the life expected of him as heir to the family business. The expansive chapter (596–645) preceding the typhoid fever, a chronicle of one of Hanno's schooldays, shows his cavalier resistance to the prevailing cult of success. His passionate commitment to the aesthetic is an intensified, creative version of his uncle Christian's attraction to the theater. Hanno's complete indifference to the Buddenbrook ethos is a psychological factor in his death, in which he "seems complicit."[16] Such a claim is supported by the concluding words to the chapter; while still eschewing direct comment, the narrator points to the decisive influence of the patient's desires at the crucial fork in the road between life and death. If he responds positively to the call of life, he may yet return, however far he has moved toward death. "Aber zuckt er zusammen vor Furcht und Abneigung bei der Stimme des Lebens, die er vernimmt, bewirkt diese Erinnerung, dieser lustige, herausfordernde Laut, dass er den Kopf schüttelt und in Abwehr die Hand hinter sich streckt, und sich vorwärts flüchtet auf dem Wege, der sich ihm zum Entrinnen eröffnet hat . . . , nein, es ist klar, dann wird er sterben." (647; But if he shudders in fear and repugnance at the voice of life that he hears, if this memory, this cheerful, challenging sound makes him shake his head and extend his hand to hold it off, to flee further along the path of escape that has opened up before him . . . no, then it is clear that he will die). The psychological dimension of Hanno's death is here unmistakably enunciated.

Hanno's death hovers in the shadowy borderlands between the somatic and the psychosomatic. In Hanno, Thomas, and Christian the interplay between the physical and the psychological is subtly illustrated. Thus Hanno's death can be attributed to the accidental swallowing of contaminated water and/or to his impulse to thanatos. In Thomas's untimely stroke too, physical elements such as the cholesterol-laden diet and sedentary lifestyle of his class and time could well play some part. Early on in the novel, at Christian's childhood indigestion, Dr. Grabow reflects on the local tendency to sudden, sometimes premature death following a heavy meal. Mann's realism motivates the inclusion of possible somatic causations of Hanno's and Thomas's death, although no doubt is left as to the underlying preponderance of the psychological. Christian, too, is later in life found to have rheumatism, which would account for some of his pain.[17]

The connections between biological events and the intervening psychosocial variables in *Buddenbrooks* are further confirmed by the contrast between the family's earlier and later generations. Most of the members of the first two generations live to a ripe old age, and exhibit no psychosomatic disorders. Well integrated into their environment, they enjoy high prestige in the city's business community and participate actively in its social round. Their lives are free of either major stresses or much imagination; one black sheep who marries beneath his station, a little flute-playing, and a modicum of piety: this is the rarely troubled tenor of the Buddenbrooks at their healthy peak.

The later generations speak through their bodies because they have been trained to utmost self-control and silence. The ethos of stoicism dictates holding one's tongue about personal problems and anxieties. This ideology is part of the general desire to make life appear pleasant. Emblematic of this is the room where the Buddenbrooks most frequently assemble, the "landscape room," whose walls are decorated with pastoral scenes reminiscent of eighteenth-century idylls. Mention of unpleasant matters is to be avoided as far as possible. Although the Buddenbrooks are often shown in animated conversation, as soon as any disagreeable, let alone menacing topic surfaces, Thomas's mother, Elisabeth, gives the categorical command "[A]ssez" (enough) that puts a peremptory stop to further discussion of the matter. The interjection of that single word, in French, is a powerful reminder of the standards of decorum in that family and that society. Such a ban inevitably results in the suppression of painful issues, and so links to the practice of keeping up appearances by masking anything that might seem offensive to the prevailing codes. From suppression and masking it is a small step to repression and conversion, with body language substituting for verbal utterance.

The dominance of polite talk about comfortable things to the exclusion of uncomfortable essentials is a recurrent feature of *Buddenbrooks*. After Tony's first divorce, for example, "Man ging behutsam umher und sprach nicht gerne 'davon' . . ." (195; They trod carefully and did not like to speak about "it" . . .). The suspension points, together with the quotation marks, while continuing the silence, invite readers to reflect on what remains unsaid. Earlier already, as Tony is trying to reach a decision about doing her duty by marrying a man she dislikes and sacrificing her love for a socially unsuitable partner, Tom, who is in a parallel situation, is on the verge of saying something and then opts for silence. "Schweigen" (not speaking) is a key term in the novel. "Sie schwiegen" (461; they were silent) about the imprisonment of Tony's son-in-law, after also maintaining silence for years about his uncouth behavior at home ("Wir haben natürlich geschwiegen"; 469). Tony's "natürlich" (naturally) projects the custom for handling the distasteful. This convention is reinforced when the narrator resorts to an impersonal construction, almost in indirect discourse, in writing of the hatred between Thomas and Christian: "Man spricht nicht davon. Man vertuscht es. Man braucht nichts davon zu wissen" (231; One does not talk about it. One keeps it in the dark. One does not need to know about it).

The many such out-of-bounds "its" that linger unvoiced among the Buddenbrooks form fertile ground for conversion disorders. For Thomas it is a relief "nichts mehr sagen zu müssen . . ." (409; not to have to say anything more . . .). Just as he retreats behind his mask, he lapses into silence: "Er sagte nichts, er sprach sich nicht aus . . ." (405; he said nothing, he did not speak his mind . . .). The suspension points in both instances suggest what might have been said, but when Tony returns to the problem, "hatte er sich in desto ablehnenderes Schweigen gehüllt" (405; he had wrapped himself in an even more resistant silence). All he does finally say is, "[I]ch wollte, wir könnten das ganz einfach ignorieren!" (405; I wish we could simply ignore it!). Tom's habitual personal silences contrast with the fluency of his public speeches in the city senate, where his eloquence wins him admiration. On the other hand, between him and his wife there are no more than minimal formal exchanges. Their marriage remains an enigma because they are never shown expressing their feelings. Tom and Gerda do

not discuss their son, let alone Tom's suspicion of her attachment to a lieu-
tenant with whom she makes music. Overwhelmed by anxieties about the
future of his business and his son as well as the possibility of scandal about
his wife, conditioned to suppress rather than to speak out, Thomas eagerly
seizes upon Schopenhauer's prospect of a future nirvana as an alluring
escape from the intolerable pressures of his earthly life.

Hanno, following his mother's lead, finds his escape in music. His
incapacity to speak is graphically brought out in the episode when the
small boy falters in his recital of a poem at the celebration of his father's
election to the senate. Openly humiliated, with tears streaming down his
face, he comes to the bitter recognition that he would never be able to
speak to people. This realization echoes his uncle Christian's declaration at
the time of his indigestion that he would never eat again. But whereas
Christian is childishly comical, Hanno is deadly earnest. His trepidation is
so intense that his voice gives out on him totally. He has no control over an
automatic bodily function. His father scornfully tells him: "Du darfst
stumm und dumm vor dich hinbrüten, dein Lebtag!" (435; You can brood
your way through your entire life, dumb and dim!). The assonance of
"stumm" and "dumm" in German is persuasive in equating the incapacity
to speak with stupidity. The irony of this pronouncement resides in the fact
that Thomas, himself remains screened behind a carefully cultivated
façade. Yet Thomas, in the third Buddenbrook generation, is still able to
don the mask and speak in public (if not in private), while Hanno, in the
fourth generation, makes no attempt at such pretense. His music teacher,
with greater insight than his father, initiates him into composition, so that
sometime later in a life that would perhaps shut his mouth tighter and
tighter, he would have the possibility of expression. Hanno, the end of the
Buddenbrooks, coincides with the end of speech.

Not all the Buddenbrooks are so taciturn. Quite the contrary: Christian and Tony are positively garrulous. Christian's interminable stream of
chatter about his physical symptoms irritates Thomas: "[S]chwatze nicht!"
(269; don't jabber!), he commands in a curt reiteration of his mother's
"assez." Christian repeatedly indulges in the most unpleasant prattling in
direct antithesis to the restraint for which Thomas strives. But although
Christian spouts volubly on his bodily condition, his discourse is remarkable for both its disjointedness and his avoidance of any expression of his
feelings except on his two or three encounters with Thomas. Significantly,
these arguments are initiated by Thomas in response to Christian's uncontrolled babbling. But Christian maintains silence about his discomfort in
the family; in this respect, indeed, he conforms to conventions, using his ill
health as a substitute outlet for emotions of hostility and estrangement
inadmissible in his environment.

Tony, too, likes to hold forth on her misfortunes. Her talk is repetitive and stereotyped because she retains a childlike naïveté despite her series of bad experiences. Her obedient recitation of the Catechism on the novel's opening page sets the pattern for her subsequent speech. She picks up phrases, for instance the recommendation of honey as a nutritious food by Morten, the medical student who is her first love, and reiterates them on later occasions. Frequently these fragments function as leitmotifs in *Buddenbrooks;* so Tony's advocacy of honey acts as an unspoken reminder of her lasting love for Morten, a love she renounced for the sake of "the family and the firm," but has neither forgotten nor overcome. She fastens on to surface detail as a displaced cipher of the strong feelings she had had; she cannot refer to Morten other than in this secret, inferential manner by invoking honey. In a way, she masks, like Tom, though much less consciously so. She also sets great store by keeping up appearances as part of the survivor's optimism, but she can do so only at the cost of not probing deeply. Her talk is often inconsequential, motivated partly by a desire to hold center stage and to bolster her self-importance as well as to submerge essential issues in mere chatter. When Tom, in a depressive mood, once confides in her, she affirms the therapeutic value of talk, but it hardly ever occurs among the Buddenbrooks. More characterstic is the dry clearing of the throat that Tony develops late in life and that is associated with her nervous stomach; it seems like a preparation for—and a thwarted alternative to—speaking.

The silences, the masks, the suppressions and repressions customary in the Buddenbrook family amount to more than failures to speak out; they connote refusals to face realities about themselves, their relationships to one another and to the world in which they live. All the major figures in the central third generation harbor a secret, and different though they are in behavior and response, they turn out to guard the same secret: their inability to uphold the ideals that this family had long cherished and represented.

Seen from this perspective, Christian, the ne'er-do-well, the invalid, the sick spot on the body of the family, emerges, with considerable irony, as the most conspicuous incarnation of the family's decline, and thus in a sense as the leading representative of his generation. His downward trajectory prefigures and parallels that of the family as a whole. By casting Christian as an aberration, by scapegoating him, the other family members, especially Thomas, try to deny their consciousness of their own demoralization. In Christian, Thomas glimpses the dreaded mirror image of himself that he has kept at bay by stringent self-discipline. For Christian exhibits "the traits [that] contribute substantially to the decline of the family" in a more open, "grotesque form"[18] than his siblings.

With his profusion of psychosomatic complaints, Christian is certainly the most obvious, though by no means the only "sick spot" in the family. On occasion he is capable of shrewd insight into others, even if we cannot ascertain the extent to which he knows himself. However, he is well able to see through his brother's façade; in a second confrontation that complements the earlier one when Thomas branded Christian as "a sick spot," Christian turns the tables in his blunt dissection of Thomas's egoistical, self-protective style:

> "Aber am schlimmsten ist das Schweigen, am schlimmsten ist es, wenn du auf etwas, was man gesagt hat, plötzlich verstummst und dich zurückziehst und jede Verantwortung ablehnst, vornehm und intakt, und den anderen hilflos seiner Beschämung überlässt. . . . Du bist ohne Mitleid und Liebe und Demut. . . . Ach!" rief er plötzlich, indem er beide Hände hinter seinen Kopf bewegte und sie dann weit vorwärts stiess, als wehrte er die ganze Welt von sich ab. . . . "Wie satt ich das alles habe, dies Taktgefühl und Feingefühl und Gleichgewicht, diese Haltung und Würde . . . wie sterbenssatt." (492–93)

> ("But the worst thing is your silence, the worst thing is when you suddenly grow mute and withdrawn in response to something that someone has said to you; you reject any responsibility, you remain elegantly uninvolved, and leave the other helplessly to his shame. . . . You are without pity or love or humility. . . . Oh!" he suddenly cried out, raising both hands behind his head and then pushing them forward as if he were distancing the whole world from himself. . . . "How sick I am of all this, this tact and delicacy and equanimity, this propriety and dignity . . . sick to death")

Christian is here not only repudiating the entire Buddenbrook ethos; he is also unmasking Thomas by spelling out the weaknesses that underlie his stance. Thomas's elegant, remote dignity stems not from strengths but from failings in his character, better concealed than Christian's evident shortcomings, yet perhaps even more damning and damaging on account of the fundamental hypocrisy. The despised, disempowered member of the family empowers himself by, for once, speaking his feelings.

The portrayal of psychosomatic disorders in *Buddenbrooks* is subtle and differentiated. Christian's flamboyant performances and constant lamentations are the extreme, blatant form. Tony's stomach complaint, though a common mode of conversion, is a more indirect way of conveying the unease beneath her determined optimism. In Thomas somatization is less immediately recognizable, partly because of the compulsive control he exerts over the image he presents to the world, but his lifelong dependence on cigarettes and his notorious nervousness indicate his need to find a compensatory outlet for repressed feelings by speaking through his body. And Hanno, who can express himself solely through music, turns his back entirely onto the world he is supposed to inherit, realizing his desire for permanent escape in death.

In conversion disorders Mann hit upon the ideal metaphor for the theme of decline. The Buddenbrooks' decline is literally embodied in their biopsychological states. The vitality of the earlier generations is in consonance with their commercial prosperity and their social security. As the rapport between self and environment becomes less spontaneous, tensions creep in. The need to keep up the appearance not only of success but also of conformity to the prevailing ethos creates ever increasing pressures. Prohibited by the creed of both their family and their cast to speak of their problems and anxieties, the later generations of Buddenbrooks speak through their bodies. Their lowered health is at once a sign and an outcome of their decline. Their flight into psychosomatic disorders provides the necessary escape from a burden they can no longer carry.

CHAPTER EIGHT

"Legs Turned to Butter"

Arthur Miller, *Broken Glass* (1994)

The body pays for the mind
—Maria Edgeworth,
The Absentee

"Her legs turned to butter, I couldn't stand her up. Kept falling around like a rag doll. I had to carry her into the house," Phillip Gellburg tells the family physician, Dr. Harry Hyman, at the opening of *Broken Glass* (20). He is describing the abrupt onset of paralysis in his wife, Sylvia, nine days previously as they were setting off down the porch steps to go to a movie. Since then she has been confined to a wheelchair or bed with no change in her disturbing state.

Dr. Hyman's explanations to Phillip, which function as the exposition to the drama, follow the medical protocol of ruling out possible diagnoses. Since Sylvia has no fever, it is not polio. In fact, "[S]he's in perfect health otherwise," Phillip proclaims (6). Dr. Hyman assures him that he and Dr. Sherman, the consultant neurologist, "can find no physical reason for her inability to walk" (15). Later he explains to Sylvia's sister, Harriet: "Her numbness is random, it doesn't follow the nerve paths; only part of the thighs are affected, part of the calves; it makes no physiological sense" (46). These inconsistencies in the clinical picture, typical of somatoform disorders, quickly lead Dr. Hyman to the conclusion that "this is a psychological condition . . . what we call an hysterical paralysis" (6). He carefully elaborates on the meaning of "hysterical," rebutting Phillip's facile designation of his wife as "crazy" (6). Her symptom denotes not a neurological disease but a signal of distress. Miller cleverly uses the doctor's opening conversations with Phillip to give the audience the necessary medical information about conversion disorders. Sylvia's paralysis conforms exactly to the criteria laid down in *DSM-IV*.[1] On this primary biological level the play is remarkably straightforward. The ready recognition of Sylvia's paralysis as a conversion disorder turns *Broken Glass* into a drama of psychological detection. What has driven this apparently healthy housewife in her mid-forties into her present invalidism?

The dismay of those around her is intensified by Sylvia's own surprising nonchalance about her disability. For in this crisis she exhibits none of the alarm that one would normally expect under such circumstances. On the contrary, "she doesn't seem all that unhappy" (23), Dr. Hyman notes, calling her stance "a funny thing" (25). Phillip goes further: "It's like she's almost . . . I don't know . . . enjoying herself. I mean in a way" (24). Her sister reiterates the same phrases: "I'll tell you something funny—to me sometimes she seems . . . I was going to say happy, but it's more like . . . I don't know . . . like this is how she wants to be. I mean since the collapse" (47). Dr. Hyman tries to confront Sylvia with the peculiarity of her situation and behavior: "[H]ere it's eleven in the morning and you're happily tucked into bed like it's midnight"; but she ignores his implied reproof, asking rather whether he is sure it is not "a virus of some kind" (62). The recurrent terms of pleasure ("happy," "enjoying") indicate that something bizarre and incongruous is occurring in Sylvia's mind. Her strange equanimity in the face of her paralysis is a classic instance of a reaction known in psychiatry as *la belle indifférence,* a relative lack of concern about the nature or implications of the symptom.[2] Equally characteristic of conversion disorder is the dependency and adoption of the sick role into which Sylvia willingly falls, abdicating her responsibility for herself and the housekeeping. The maid comes in the morning to help her bathe, later her sister cares for her, while the onus for much of the housework—shopping, cooking, laundry—falls onto her husband. Despite the drawbacks of her paralysis, Sylvia obviously derives secondary gain from it by becoming the center of solicitous attention from various quarters. "Just trying to get out of doing the dishes" (60), Dr. Hyman ventures with pseudo-jocularity.

Doubling as the voice of both medical science and puzzled spectators, Dr. Hyman summarizes the central enigma of *Broken Glass* when he says: "We have a strong healthy woman, who has no physical ailment, and suddenly can't stand on her legs. Why?" (18). The search for the answer to that question propels the play and maintains the suspense. For Sylvia's paralysis is the catalyst that destabilizes the Gellburgs' marriage. Sylvia's appearance on stage either in a wheelchair or in bed is a graphic visual representation of her disability; at the same time, as she speaks through her body, it is a metaphor for her inner, unconscious perception of where she stands in life—or rather, of where and what she literally cannot *stand.* Her physical paralysis represents the externalization of the emotional impasse in which she is trapped. What then has impelled this woman, described in the stage directions as "buxom, capable, and warm" (30) and by her husband as "level-headed" (20), to this extreme?

Having formulated the question "Why?", Dr. Hyman wants to try to answer it by acting as detective/therapist, although he admits not only that he barely knows his way around psychiatry (27) but also shows a certain prejudice against it by referring to "that whole psychiatric rigmarole" (17). He wants to spare Sylvia that kind of experience in the belief that "you get further faster, sometimes, with a little common sense and some plain human sympathy" (17). His remarks have to be read in the context of the time of the play's action in the late 1930s, when the "psychiatric rigmarole" would probably have meant protracted psychoanalysis, which then had many followers, yet aroused the skepticism of such advocates of "common sense" as Dr. Hyman. In keeping with his creed of sense combined with sensibility, his manner is direct and down-to-earth; he repeatedly speaks of his wish to "talk turkey" (17), and urges Phillip to "try to face the facts" (18).

Dr. Hyman's motivation for taking on a case that "fascinates" (27) him is manifold. He wants to help a patient in trouble; he admires her for having "a lot of courage" (9), and he has the incentive of loyalty to a family with whom he has a long-standing association. He also sees in Sylvia a professional challenge, an opportunity to prove his own abilities by not simply "shipping all the hard cases to specialists" (27). His pride and his self-worth are at stake in his desire to solve a perplexing medicopsychological mystery. Despite his lack of formal training in psychiatry, he proves well qualified to handle this case: he is shown to be a fine psychologist, a shrewd observer with sound instincts, a perceptive listener, and in command of sufficient human experience and medical knowledge to probe the problem with acuity and insight. Right away he has "the feeling she may be afraid" of annoying Phillip by talking about certain things, and he floats the possibility of "a sexual disability" as a common root for this type of paralysis. He seems to possess greater familiarity with psychiatry than he claims. With a mixture of observation and intuition, his hypothesis foreshadows some of the revelations that will come later in the play.

But the action unfolds by a roundabout route. As in all good detective stories, a red herring first creates a distraction and a detour before more valid answers to the question "Why?" gradually emerge.

The initially dominant supposition, voiced by several characters, connects Sylvia's impairment to her being "very upset" (11) about recent events in Germany. In the last days of November 1938, the time of Crystal Night the newspapers are full of the outrages against Jews. Dr. Hyman raises this topic in his conversation with Phillip in the opening scene; Phillip seems unconcerned, excusing his detachment by the extremely long hours he spends at the office. But soon after he tries to persuade Sylvia that "this whole Nazi business" is the cause of her paralysis, since Dr. Hyman "claims that being very frightened could do it" (40). Phillip endorses this view with enthusiasm by emphasizing how Sylvia "scares herself to death" (19) with the horrifying pictures that should, in his opinion, not be published at all. Her abnormal excitement at the pictures and reports in the newspapers is noted by her sister too: "So why are you interested in that? What business of yours is that?" (33). Sylvia's perturbation is in glaring contrast to both her indifference to her paralysis and to her husband's lack of interest in the outrageous events in Germany.

The impact of Crystal Night is thematized in the play's title, *Broken Glass*. Through the repeated references to Sylvia's fixation on the newspapers, the audience is led to believe that her paralysis has its origins in this fright. Sylvia's evident distress further supports this interpretation: "What is going to become of us?" she exclaims; in even more acute agitation she screams: "This is an *emergency!* What if they kill those children! Where is Roosevelt? Where is England? Somebody should do something before they murder us all!" (107). Her reaction might indeed seem to be excessive (except in hindsight). Her use here of "us" shows her identification with those under attack. One of the old men in the newspaper strikes her as the "spitting image" of her grandfather with the same "bent sidepiece" (33) to his eyeglasses. Her emotional vehemence about happenings in Europe is in stark antithesis to her insouciance about the upheaval in her own home. That the trauma of the broken glass might be the psychosocial trigger to her disorder is made to seem a possibility.

Sylvia's anxieties appear much less far-fetched in light of the rampant anti-Semitism of the 1930s, which historians see as its "worst period."[3] Societal changes in the 1920s and the Great Depression "intensified and exacerbated attitudes that had already manifested themselves earlier. These hostile feelings coalesced from the 1920s through 1945 at such an accelerated pace that many Jews thought that what happened in Hitler's Germany might very well occur in the United States as well."[4] Although the social historian Leonard Dinnerstein dismisses such ideas as "preposterous . . . fantasies," he concedes that they "fueled fear and the increased incidence of bigotry and discrimination whipped the Jewish people in America into a frenzy of panic" (212). These words confirm the prevalence of Sylvia's responses. While she is the exception in *Broken Glass* in sensing a direct, personal threat in the newspaper reports from Germany, she is neither alone nor unreasonable in the wider social context. The portents were ominous. The German-American Bund, heavily influenced by the Fascist example in Central Europe, was foremost among scores of similar anti-Semitic groups that sprang up at this period, inspired by the Nazi persecution. Roosevelt's New Deal was nicknamed the "Jew Deal" because of the number of Jews in the federal government.[5] Father Charles E. Coughlin's sensationalist, inflammatory weekly radio sermons in the 1930s disseminated a strain of irrational hatred. As Myron Scholnick documents, "starting in 1933, the noise level of Jew-baiting in the United States rose to unprecedented heights" (62).

Nor was it merely a matter of "noise" and rhetoric. Discrimination against Jews in the job market was a grave problem, aggravated by the high levels of unemployment during the Depression. Dinnerstein points out that "some chose to deal with the problem by changing their names and trying by other means to hide their origins" (213). This is the tactic adopted by Phillip. His calculated effort to distance himself from his Jewishness is a central motif in *Broken Glass*. In the opening scene he takes offense when Margaret, Dr. Hyman's wife and receptionist, twice addresses him as "Goldberg" instead of "Gellburg." The rarity of "Gellburg" and the commonness of "Goldberg," together with Phillip's irritation, immediately arouses the suspicion that he had changed his name. Phillip links his name to his family's alleged roots in Finland but subsequently lets out that his parents were from "Poland somewhere or Russia" (24). In his name and background he deliberately cultivates a non-Jewish semblance. He boasts of being "the only Jew [who] ever worked for Brooklyn Guarantee in their whole history" (22) as well as "the only Jew" who has set foot on the deck of the boat that is the prized possession of his immediate superior in the bank, Mr. Case (21). He takes even greater pride in "the captain" (35), as he calls his son Jerome, who is making a career in the army. This is the one subject on which Sylvia openly disagrees with her husband, lamenting: "Who goes into the army? Men who can't do anything else" (36). Phillip, on the other hand, asserts: "I wanted people to see that a Jew doesn't have to be a lawyer or a doctor or a businessman" (36). "He could be the first Jewish general in the United States Army" (37), he adds. Phillip overrides his wife's objections in steering their son into the army. He does not seem to resent the fact that Jerome would never have got into West Point without Mr. Case's connections. He even tolerates without demur Mr. Case's reiterated rather contemptuous phrase "one of you people" (56).

Phillip's flight from, almost abnegation, of his Jewishness is in part prudent self-protection. But his need to brag about being the only Jewish employee in his bank suggests an undercurrent of insecurity. The excessively long hours he puts in at the office project an overzealousness that is a bulwark against the stress he experiences in his dread of criticism.

Nonetheless, he is peremptorily fired as a result of a bad decision he has recommended on the basis of information from a business contact, Allan Kershowitz, "also a Jew" (118). More damaging than his miscalculation itself is Phillip's provocative behavior toward Mr. Case; incensed at his own fallibility, he attributes to others base motives for precipitating his downfall. Because he projects an edited (if not a false) persona, he suspects others of a similar deviousness, thereby creating a climate of mistrust. He is a man with a chip on his shoulder, who is trying hard to hide both that chip and its origins. His posturing is well illustrated in his habit of invariably wearing black, which gives him a sinister appearance but serves primarily as a mask. Having started in business at age twenty-two, he wanted to look older, he explains; "[I]t gives you authority?" Dr. Hyman proposes (23). Phillip's black clothing is the manifestation, at once visible and metaphoric, of his attempt to construct a self other than what he really is: not pronouncedly Jewish, but strong, authoritative, and successful.

Phillip's dissociation from his Jewishness also shows up the mean streak in his character. He may not, as Dr. Hyman puts it, "like being Jewish," indeed "he'd rather not be one" (49); he may also incline toward being a Republican, asking with scornful irony whether "the Torah says a Jew has to be a Democrat" (12). "I don't run with the crowd," he asserts (12). However, not running with the crowd entails a perverse anti-Semitism on his part. He is critical of the refugees from Poland and Russia as "pushy," and even more so of the German Jews who "won't take an ordinary good job . . . ; it's got to be pretty high up in the firm, or they're insulted. And they don't even speak English" (12). Phillip's own vulnerability to job loss probably influences his prejudice against new immigrants, whom he may see as potential rivals for employment. By emphasizing their defects, he is at pains to separate his superior self from them. Yet his anti-Semitism and his arrogance cast a bad light on him.

Phillip's harsh attitude is thrown into relief by Dr. Hyman's greater tolerance. He has himself been the object of anti-Semitism because American medical schools "have quotas on Jews" (68). Rather than wait for years and risk still not getting in, he took his M.D. in Heidelberg. He cherishes happy memories of his student days and has not developed any complexes. "I never pretended I wasn't Jewish," he "coldly" tells Phillip (129). Nor has he changed his name, an archetypally Jewish name, not least through its resonance of the derogatory "Hymietown" for New York. Admittedly, being in an independent profession as a physician, he is less exposed to anti-Semitism than Philip, an employee. Dr. Hyman's attitude to the current political developments is halfway between Phillip's and Sylvia's: he does not, like Phillip, ignore the threat, for he finds "this Adolf Hitler very disturbing" (10); on the other hand, he does not panic, like Sylvia.

Another "why?" arises at this point. If Sylvia's fears at Crystal Night are not the ulterior cause of her paralysis, as eventually turns out, why give it so much attention in the first part of the play? A number of possible answers to this question overlap. First, the events of Crystal Night firmly anchor the action in the sociopolitical situation of 1938; the widespread anxieties among American Jews evoked by this escalation of persecution is a fitting context (if not an explanation) for Sylvia's frightened state. So anti-Semitism is an important "intermediate variable" for the formation of the conversion disorder in *Broken Glass*.[6] Second, the response to Crystal Night is a means of disclosing the unpleasantness in Phillip's character. Already in his initial interview with Dr. Hyman he does not come across as a likable personality. Incidentally, it is Phillip who forcefully presses the interpretation that it is the pictures of the violence against Jews in Germany that have elicited Sylvia's paralysis. In retrospect, this view turns out to be a diversionary tactic on Phillip's part, another facet of his self-protective stance. Finally, and most important, the broken glass is the occasion for the outbreak of Sylvia's paralysis because it raises her consciousness of her Jewishness, and therefore brings into the open the crucial discord between her and her husband. Once this initial wedge has been driven in, the whole marriage begins to unravel. The public ferment on the European scene is correlative to the private turmoil in the Gellburgs' home. The social destabilization serves as a frame to the psychological disarray; Sylvia's outer and inner worlds are falling apart to a degree she can no longer *stand*.

The broken glass of the Crystal Night can also be linked to the glass broken as part of the Jewish wedding ceremony. That ritual is intended as a reminder, even at the happiest moments, of the dark sides of Jewish history, especially the destruction of the temple in Jerusalem in A.D. 71. Broken glass is thus endowed in this play with both a traditional and a personal meaning; in Sylvia's mind it represents at once metonymically and metaphorically her splintered marriage as well as the political threat. Just as the Jews went into exile after the destruction of the temple, so Phillip and Sylvia are in figurative exile from each other and from their own selves.

Broken Glass thus opens up a series of layers as the secrets behind Sylvia's paralysis are exposed one by one. The surface disparity between her and Phillip's reactions to the reports from Germany leads toward the deeper issues that fester in this marriage and so to the emotions that underlie the conversion disorder. Memory is created bit by bit through the medium of illness as the past is uncovered and rewritten.

To what extent are Sylvia and Phillip aware of the problems they have refused to confront individually and jointly? Toward the end of the play both admit their sense of feeling somehow lost in their lives, as Phillip says: "I don't know where I am" (128) and Sylvia, "I can't find myself in my life" (136). But these avowals come very late, after twenty or so years of denial and evasion. Sylvia and Phillip bear out Barbour's observation about a "fascinating aspect of the conversion process," namely "that parts are acted, a drama unfolds, a game is played, but none of the players is fully aware of the process."[7] Barbour believes that "the patient does not seem to know much about what might be going on at an emotional level. But this patient is actually an alternate personality dissociated from the physically well but emotionally distressed real person who does know. The 'sick patient' is doing the talking, but the real person is watching the interaction silently and unobtrusively in the background" (193).

This scenario is apposite to Sylvia, who repeatedly replies to Dr. Hyman's probing questions with a blunt "I don't know." Asked by her husband whether she is afraid of something, as the doctor has suggested, she responds twice in rapid succession with that same phrase. On the conscious level she really seems not to know, for she assures Dr. Hyman: "I would tell you if I knew" (63). The doctor continues to urge her on, for he realizes how imperative it is for her to recognize and acknowledge the truth: "Sylvia, I know you know more than you're saying" (68) until she concedes: "I have no word for it, I don't know what I'm saying, it's like . . . *She presses her chest.* —something alive, like a child almost, except it's a very dark thing . . . and it frightens me!" (69). It is after this initial confession that Dr. Hyman applies the word "secret" (70) to the things she needs to tell him. Whether these secret things are consciously known to her remains unclear to the doctor—and probably to her too. Dr. Hyman confides to his wife: "Margaret—she *knows* something! I don't know what it is, and she may not either—but I tell you it's real" (85). The psychological damage wreaked in the long term by the tension between knowing and not knowing, especially not *wanting* to know, is a cardinal theme of *Broken Glass*.

In not wanting to know, Sylvia and Phillip are alike, though for different reasons. In her case it is largely a matter of repression, stemming from her conviction that her situation is beyond redemption. She has acted out the role that Phillip and societal expectations in the 1930s imposed on her as submissive wife and mother. Sylvia's story emerges in haphazard snippets from her conversations with her sister and mainly with Dr. Hyman. The first hint of the resentment she harbors is introduced quite casually as she insists to her sister that she must send her son to college: "If I'd had a chance to go to college, I'd have had a whole different life" (32). Sylvia's frustration at the opportunities she has been denied is here uttered in unmistakable terms. The conversion of her mental anguish into physical pain is modeled in her complaint at this point of "a deep, terrible aching"

(31) in her entire being. As the eldest in the family, she had the duty of looking after her sisters from an early age onward and so never enjoyed the freedom of, for instance, going to the beach with her peers. In her first job, as head bookkeeper at a firm in Long Island City, she met Phillip, married him, and bore a son. The outer story of her life is scant and uneventful.

Her more complex inner story opens up slowly at Dr. Hyman's incessant prompting. He notices how her eyes show fear when he asks her whether they can talk about Phillip. In the ensuing conversation Sylvia is very ambivalent, changing her answers, changing the subject, wanting to speak because it makes her feel "hopeful" (66), yet at the same time clearly exhibiting anxiety. She does disclose one central source of strife in the marriage: that she enjoyed being in business but Phillip did not want her to work after the birth of their son. This conflict is the subject of the first major confrontation between husband and wife near the close of the play. Sharp resentment still festers on both sides, more than twenty years after the original clash. Sylvia's animosity toward her husband is compounded retrospectively by a burst of anger against herself for having given in to his authority. Phillip, in turn, recalls his dismay at her sudden unwillingness "to keep the house anymore" and her preference for going to business. The phrase "to keep the house" can have a dual meaning: literally it denotes simply to do the housekeeping, but figuratively it can connote the sense of disempowerment, indeed oppression, that Sylvia felt at being kept in the house. She becomes de facto captive to Phillip. When he makes the accusation "You never forgave me, Sylvia" (113), she does not negate his contention. In one sense, therefore, her paralysis represents a partial wish fulfillment in releasing her from the housekeeping to which she had been condemned. But she continues to be deprived of the satisfying occupation outside the home essential to her self-esteem.

In probing her paralysis, Dr. Hyman astutely asks: "[W]hy are you cut off from yourself?" (68). The question straddles the symptom and its cause. One reason why she is cut off from herself is because she could or would not assert herself against Phillip, and consequently has been frustrated in her wish to work outside the home, an activity from which she derived respect, self-respect, and a certain independence. She wants to forget, that is, cut off from herself not only the actual loss of work that was meaningful to her but also the memory of her own incapacity to stand up against her husband. By being made to keep the house, she is also cut off from using her high intelligence. Harriet cites her husband's opinion that "God gave Sylvia all the brains" (49). Dr. Hyman, too, describes her as "a remarkably well-informed woman," a comment that provokes from Phillip a comment both revealing and indirectly self-incriminating: "That's practically why we got together in the first place. I don't exaggerate, if Sylvia was a man she could have run the Federal Reserve. You could talk to Sylvia like you talk to a man" (14). She had on occasion had to explain the firm's accounts to Phillip, who quips: "I fell in love with her figures" (49). Yet Sylvia's intellectual abilities, at first a source of her attractiveness, clearly posed a threat to him over the years. Margaret, who is credited by Dr. Hyman with having "a very good diagnostic sense" (72), immediately typecasts Phillip as "a dictator" and "one miserable little pisser" (26). Harriet divulges that he once threw a steak at Sylvia because it was overdone. By the end of the first act, a negative picture of the Gellburgs' marriage has been formed in the audience's mind, with Phillip as the villain controlling Sylvia. Her paralysis appears as a form of rebellion, even revenge.

But this explanation, like that devolving from the broken glass of the Crystal Night, also proves to be only a partial one. For in the second act, further layers are peeled away as the grounds for Phillip's anger, furtiveness, and posturing are exposed.

Phillip knows only too well what he does not want to know, and so does Sylvia, although both have banned the subject in a consensual censorship. What is more, his relatives suspect as well; Harriet reports the local men's gossip to Dr. Hyman: "[H]e got so mad . . . because he couldn't, you know . . ." (33). Apart from Harriet's insinuation, "that" and "it" (42), while mentioned in the first act of *Broken Glass* already, appear solely as taboo topics between Phillip and Sylvia. When Dr. Hyman early on brings up "a sexual disability" as a frequent causality in cases such as Sylvia's, Phillip is described in the stage directions as "*hostile,*" "*flushed,*" and "*relieved to be off the other subject*" (18–19) when talk turns to Crystal Night. For him the broken glass is a godsend that he can exploit as a convenient screen for the deeper and more personal problem that he wants at all costs to keep hidden.

Not until a very late stage in the drama is Phillip's impotence brought directly into the open. It dates back to the time after Jerome's birth when Sylvia wanted to go back to work and Phillip refused to let her. She never forgave him, he claims:

> *She evades his gaze*
> GELLBURG: So whenever I . . . when I started to touch you, I felt that.
> SYLVIA: You felt what?
> GELLBURG: That you didn't want me to be the man here. And then, on top of that when you didn't want any more children . . . everything made me just dried up. (113–14)

The disempowerment is thus in a curious way mutual and interdependent; when Phillip debars Sylvia from work, she rejects him conjugally. Phillip's physical impotence is the countersymbol to the image he has tried to nurture, the stealthy, long concealed cipher for the hollowness of his façade. In its inauthenticity his outer social persona coincides with his inner, psychological state. He is unable to *be* what he wishes to *appear.*

Since he has the prerogative, according to the conventions of 1938, to be the dominant partner in the marriage, Phillip projects the blame onto Sylvia. He accuses her of having unmanned him by wanting herself "to be the man here." In his mind, for a woman to work outside the home is tantamount to assuming a male role. He is, therefore, convinced that "this whole thing is against me" (75) in further unmanning him by shifting the womanly domestic chores onto him. Here Phillip is more than just grossly domineering; he sounds almost paranoic as he attributes to Sylvia a calculated aim in her paralysis. His subjective, probably guilt-ridden, distorted "perception and cognition"[8] of the problem is revealed in his reaction to Sylvia's symptom. In his rage and blindness, he cannot recognize that his impotence is another kind of paralysis, virtually the equivalent to hers. Both Phillip and Sylvia are inhibited in vital physical functions by the effect of long unacknowledged psychological inhibitions. The subconscious impact of these forces surfaces in Phillip's wish fantasy of making love to Sylvia and in her anxiety dream of being violated by Phillip—and the Nazis. The cessation of their sexual relations bears out Deutsch's contention that "motor paralysis is a form of defense against a certain action which should have been carried out in a given situation but which has been repressed."[9]

This repression leads to the mendacity of their marriage at both the sexual and the human, communicative levels and is the secret that ties this couple to each other, like Thérèse and Laurent in *Thérèse Raquin.* Husband and wife are bound in a love-hate relationship through this shared secret about which they can barely speak. While they have some partial, intuitive realization of its significance, they remain entrenched in a defensive denial and locked into an ominous, destructive silence. Whereas Phillip can find some escape in his work (hence his long hours at the office), for Sylvia, stuck in the house, the only way out of her impasse lies in her paralysis, which finally brings the situation to a head.

The nature of the relationship between the Gellburgs is vividly illustrated by a small, seemingly humorous incident. When Phillip is advised by Dr. Hyman to give Sylvia "a lot of loving" (26), he brings her a gift in a small paper bag: sour pickles from a deli she used to like. The incident is on the surface comical, yet at a deeper level pathetic in the light it sheds on Phillip's emotional sterility. The choice precisely of sour pickles as a token of tenderness is a tragicomic symbol of the souredness of his affective capacity. The detail eventually takes on added significance as denoting the atrophied state of Phillip's heart, that is, as a metaphoric prefiguration of his physical condition. The episode can be extended to Sylvia too; a sour pickle is inadequate nourishment for her emotional starvation. Her paralysis is the physical manifestation of her frustrated feelings.

The discord in the Gellburg marriage is accentuated by the contrast with the other couple depicted in *Broken Glass*. Harry and Margaret Hyman represent the diametric opposite to Phillip and Sylvia in their vigor and above all in their openness with each other. In a continuation of the play's titular metaphor, Margaret tells her husband: "You don't realize how transparent you are. You're a pane of glass" (84). The word "pane" denotes intactness, in contradistinction to "broken." Harry's Jewishness is, as he puts it, "not an obsession" (129) for him; he is self-accepting, and what is more, able to adjust his heritage to suit his own tastes. As against Phillip's somber garb, Harry often appears in sportswear because he goes riding every afternoon. Ironically, the sedentary, cautious, pale Phillip, prim, proper, and hyperconservative, conforms more closely to the traditional image of the Jew than the "healthy, rather handsome" (7) outdoorsman, Harry. He has also had the courage to follow his inclinations by marrying out, a more daring step at that time when intermarriage was less common than it has since become. In answer to Phillip's blunt—and rude—question: "[H]ow'd you come to marry a shiksa?" Harry is forthright and unapologetic: "We were thrown together when I was interning, and we got very close, and . . . well she was a good partner, she helped me, and still does. And I loved her" (129). The marriage is shown, in a romanticized aura, as a happy, loving partnership with an abundance of easy, playful affection, and shared pleasures. Margaret is "lusty, energetic" (3), an enthusiastic gardener, with a tendency to be outspoken. "She chew your ear off?" Harry asks Phillip, yet he does so "chuckling" (7) with a jovial forebearance of his wife's manner. He respects the kindness and capacity for understanding beneath her occasionally brusque exterior. Their relationship is one of reciprocal trust and open communication.

The social context formed by Harry and Margaret, and to a lesser extent by Mr. Case, is important as the frame for the exploration of the psychological difficulties that have led to Sylvia's paralysis and Phillip's impotence. Margaret is the foil to Sylvia just as Harry is to Phillip. To the social pairing of Jew/non-Jew and the biological opposition of sick/healthy must be added the psychological dimension of repressed/open. Margaret's outspokenness is at one end of this spectrum along with her non-Jewishness and her ebullient robustness. She is idealized as a character free of inner conflicts.

Dr. Hyman is subject to even greater idealization as the stereotypical understanding family doctor in the old tradition. He has made his peace with being Jewish, enjoys good health, and speaks with as much candor as is compatible with the decorous limits of tact predicated by his profession. His capacity for psychological insight into his patients enables him to help them to a significant degree in a very personal style. However, his competence in dealing with a psychosomatic disorder seems to be an anachronism. In 1938 a family practitioner was hardly likely to have much awareness of psychosomatics at a period when medicine was resolutely somatic. Dunbar's *Emotions and Bodily Changes* had just appeared in 1935. It was not until the 1950s, following the publication of Alexander's *Psychosomatic Medicine,* that the concept of psychosomatic conversion came to be more widely diffused. It is well to recall that Dr. Grabow in *Buddenbrooks* has no idea how to diagnose Christian's symptoms, let alone how to deal with them. The position of Roger Chillingworth in *The Scarlet Letter* is quite different, for he works in the context of humoral medicine, which acknowledged the symbiosis of mind and body. There is no hint in *Broken Glass* that Dr. Hyman had read Freud or was even acquainted with his ideas, yet he immediately posits a possible sexual factor in the etiology of Sylvia's paralysis. In the last resort, his power stems less from theoretical medical knowledge than from sheer force of personality, experience, and intuition.

Dr. Hyman becomes the instrument for Sylvia's release from silence. He can manage the case so well for two reasons. First, as he explains to Phillip, he has "this unconventional approach to illness. Especially where the mental element is involved. I believe we get sick in twos and threes and fours, not alone as individuals" (25). This statement of Dr. Hyman's medical philosophy accounts for his preference for family practice because he envisages disorders, particularly those with a psychological component, not as encapsulated entities limited to the sufferer but as expressions of a wider dis-ease that may stem from and certainly affects a broader circle. Accordingly, Dr. Hyman wants to know his patients in twos and threes and fours, not just as isolated individuals. This essentially psychosocial concept of illness is closely akin to Engel's biopsychosocial model. It is also one determinant of his decision to take on this case himself rather than refer Sylvia to a psychiatrist, who would not be so well acquainted with her social and family context.

The second reason for Dr. Hyman's success with Sylvia stems from the trust and familiarity long established between this doctor and this patient, that lead to the speedy consolidation of a therapeutic alliance. Starved of sex and affection in her marriage, Sylvia is strongly attracted to Dr. Hyman. The tone between them is plainly flirtatious: Sylvia "*has a certain excitement at seeing him*" (60), she "*instantly smiles*" and "*holds out a hand to him,"* saying: "I'm so glad you've come" (94); he notices that her hair is done differently and that she is wearing perfume. The stage directions leave no doubt about the sexual nature of her feelings for him; after Dr. Hyman has affectionately kissed her on the cheek on taking leave, Sylvia, stretched out on the bed, *"lets her knees spread apart"* (70). Later, she takes the initiative as *"she draws him to her and kisses him on the mouth"* (99). Without ever transgressing the boundaries of propriety, the doctor builds on her attraction to him to bring her gradually to voice what had long remained unsaid. He uses both persuasion in urging her "to have more confidence, . . . in general, in life, in people" (105), and suggestion: "I know you want to tell me something and I don't know how to get it out of you" (63). In order to diminish her resistance and to obviate any sense of guilt she may have at speaking about matters hitherto carefully concealed, Dr. Hyman tells her that he has learned "that these kinds of symptoms come from very deep in the mind" (96). This assurance that her paralysis springs from the unconscious and is therefore beyond her control absolves Sylvia from responsibility for her impairment.

Through talking to Dr. Hyman, Sylvia finds release and recovery. This treatment is obviously a "talking cure," and as such it has special meaning in a play whose main theme is the atrophy of intimate communication. "Talk" is a key word that recurs constantly in *Broken Glass.* Phillip is immediately written off by Margaret as "not much of a talker" (6) when he stonewalls her efforts at pleasant conversation by his lapidary replies. Dr. Hyman finds him "not an easy man to talk to" (17), for he does not willingly listen to what others have to say. In order to cover up his insecurity and uphold his facade, Phillip has enclosed himself in a cocoon of rebarbative silence and condescension. He talks to his relatives, Harriet complains, as if they have "four legs and long ears" (48). Phillip has isolated himself into a haughty aloofness that molds his attitude to his wife too. So Sylvia, Dr. Hyman believes, has become afraid to talk. The absence of honest talk in the Gellburgs' marriage is at the heart of their difficulties, denials, and consequent repressions. All the major issues are out of bounds: "that" and "it" are certainly unmentionables; the choice of career for their son is not open to discussion; Sylvia's anxieties about Crystal Night meet with snubs and rebukes. She urgently needs to vent her feelings, and, in the face of the failure of normal communication, can do so only through her body. Her paralysis bespeaks of a distress she cannot utter verbally.

Dr. Hyman's persistent, gentle probing induces her to find the liberating words. At first, she backs off, like Phillip, behind an acquired habit of avoidance. But Dr. Hyman will not allow himself to be easily defeated; by dint of perseverance, kindness, and the "human sympathy" he extends to her, he breaks through her resistance. She begs him to talk to her, and eventually discovers that she for her part "can talk to him" (110). The psychotherapeutic transference is greatly facilitated by her personal attraction to him. She acknowledges that "after a while" in the marriage, she had not been able "to find a true word to put in [her] mouth" (122). It is this cumulative silence of repression that is the primary basis of her conversion disorder.

By learning to talk, to name her feelings, to identify her desires, to voice her distress, Sylvia attains the capacity for self-assertiveness necessary to "face the facts" and find her life. Previously she had been "here for my mother's sake, and Jerome's sake, and everybody's sake except mine" (44). With Dr. Hyman's encouragement and support, she openly challenges and defies Phillip through her determination "to say anything I want to" (112). Despite Phillip's weeping and threats, she *wants* to know "what I did with my life! Out of ignorance. Out of not wanting to shame you in front of other people. A whole life. Gave it away like a couple of pennies—I took better care of my shoes. *Turns to him.*—You want to talk about it now? Take me seriously, Phillip. What happened? I know it's all you ever thought about, isn't that true? *What happened?* Just so I'll know" (112). To express in this way the anger she has bottled up within herself for so many years is an essential preliminary to confronting her marital situation. The veritable explosion of her resentment in these staccato exclamations is the verbal equivalent to the shock created by the shattered fragments of broken glass in Germany. Her final startling breakthrough to candid self-knowledge occurs when she does forgive Phillip and also accepts her own shared coresponsibility for the broken glass of her life: "I'm not blaming you, Phillip. The years I wasted I know I threw away myself. I think I always knew I was doing it but I couldn't stop it" (136). The dissipation of the secret she has withheld from herself is the harbinger to healing. Once she can openly speak out about her distress, it no longer has to be converted into a symbolic paralysis. Even though she maintains near the end of the play: "There's nothing I know now that I didn't know twenty years ago. I just didn't say it" (121), the damage to her was done by the repression, the pretense, the evasiveness, the self-coercion and self-censorship as her subconscious rage was ultimately turned inward against herself. The reticence that was meant to have a self-protective function has acted as a noxious chronic poison in Sylvia until it finally could no longer be contained and broke out in a physical form.

In this psychodrama about the attenuation of talk, body language assumes heightened significance as the carrier of meanings. Sylvia's paralysis is the prime but by no means the sole example. Gestures and vocal tone, laid out in the stage directions, represent involuntary expressions of concealed emotions. The prominence of body language immediately becomes apparent in the opening interaction between Phillip and Margaret where his tension and discomfort are set off against her relaxed, easy style. So Phillip's manner conveys "*a faint reprimand*" (3), "*a barely hidden boast,*" "*a certain amused loftiness*" (4), "*an overtone of protest of some personal victimization*" (6), and he shows "*a purse-mouthed smile*" (7). By contrast, Margaret "*laughs in a burst*" (4), tries to "*charm him to his ease*" (5), and, though she is "*defeated*" (5) by his stubborn gruffness, emits another "*burst of laughter*" as she leaves "*with a little wave*" (7). Phillip's stiff posture ("*tense,*" "*in perfect stillness, legs crossed*" [3]) and his black clothing indicate his constraint. Even allowing for the natural element of anxiety as he awaits the doctor to discuss his wife's paralysis, Phillip's body language as much as his clipped utterances characterize him as a troubled person, accustomed to fending others off through aggressive/defensive behavior.

Throughout *Broken Glass* Miller, like Ibsen and Strindberg, acts as narrator through the medium of the stage directions, often by describing body language and occasionally by naming feelings. The characters' interactions are seen primarily from an external gaze, as they would be by an audience in the theater. Speech tends to be more terse than in the expansive genre of narrative, and there is no interior monologue to give access to private thoughts. Indeed, *Broken Glass* favors a distinctive sparseness. The action is limited in time to the last days of November 1938 and in location to three places: Dr. Hyman's office, the bedroom of the Gellburg home, and Stanton Case's office. None of these is in any way described; on the contrary, as in French seventeenth-century drama, the outer scene is quite unspecific, and for the same purpose, namely, to direct the spotlight to the site of the real action within the protagonists' minds. In their indication of veiled feelings rather than actual movements, the stage directions reinforce the play's status as a psychodrama.

As such, *Broken Glass* is at once realistic and ritualistic, signifying on the overt and the symbolical level. Generally, its realism is to the fore, for instance in the colloquial speech patterns with broken sentences and much rapid repartee, the attention to such details as clothing, and above all the very penetrating delineation of a spectrum of individuals. Its complementary ritualistic facet is most conspicuous in the recurrence of the lone cellist playing a simple tune that introduces nine of the eleven scenes. He is absent before the two scenes (act 2, scenes 3 and 4) that depict Phillip's heart attack. He seems to evoke a certain wistfulness reminiscent perhaps of the cello solo in Bruch's *Kol Nidrei*. The solemnity of the Kol Nidrei service on the eve of the Day of Atonement, the climax of the Jewish New Year holy days, is elegiac in its review of past times; it is a day of self-scrutiny, reckoning, and avowal of sins. But this holiest of days also turns toward the future in the resolve to make amends in a new start. So the cellist can be seen as relevant to those parts of the play concerned with Sylvia, and not to those about Phillip.

Phillip makes far less progress than Sylvia in emerging from his self-created prison. Since Dr. Hyman perceives patients as sickening in twos and threes, he recognizes the need to attend to Phillip too because of the couple's codependency. But the therapeutic alliance between the two men never attains the intensity or effectiveness of that between Dr. Hyman and Sylvia. Phillip remains laconic and guarded until after his first heart attack. This physical shock makes a deep impact on him in inducing him to think about himself more honestly and reassess his life as it moves to its close. His increased frankness toward himself is marked by a growing willingness to speak. By the end of the play he lets the thoughts and memories racing through his mind tumble out without his previous cautious censorship. He realizes that his attempts "to disappear into the goyim" (130), to cite the doctor's phrase, had failed, and that his true function at the bank had been precisely as the Jew to do the dirty work: "You got some lousy rotten job to do, get Gellburg, send in the Yid" (125). He identifies himself here not merely as a Jew but with the derogatory word "Yid." When Phillip falls to his hands and knees in front of Mr. Case, his posture is reminiscent of that of the humiliated Jews in Germany, so that he comes indirectly to be associated with them. When he reaffirms his Jewishness, he recalls with sentimental nostalgia a shopping expedition in the early phase of the marriage when "I felt so at home and happy there that day, a street full of Jews, one Moses after the other" (127–28). He gives up projecting a self-image as the "Rock of Gibraltar" (122), a strong man of great independence, and confesses instead that he had been "more afraid than I looked" (137). However, whether he can forgive himself "and the Jews" (135), as Dr. Hyman advises, remains an open question. The secret of his self-hatred has been exposed, but the self-hatred itself not excised. When Sylvia reassures him, after he has expressed surprise that she married him, "A Jew can have a Jewish face," he still retorts: "I can't help my thoughts" (114).

The attempt to forgive and to be more open comes too late in Phillip's life. For years he has been burdened by the guilty secret of his impotence as well as anger against the Jews, the non-Jews, and most of all against himself. It is not surprising that he suffers a heart attack at his office after his spectacular outbreak of fury about the collusion with Allan Kershowitz of which he thinks he is suspected. Phillip's collapse is sudden and dramatic, but well prepared throughout the play in the many references to his declining, strained health. "You don't look well" (54), Mr. Case tells him; he loses weight, sighs frequently, and is visibly tense. Above all, his impotence, in Sylvia's opinion, "tortures him, it's like a snake eating into his heart" (103). This image vividly captures the harm done to his heart by psychological stress. The same confluence of the psychological with the physical occurs when Phillip, at the very end, begs Sylvia, in another telling image, not to blame him anymore: "I feel I did this to you! That's the knife in my heart" (137). His reiterated fear that Sylvia's new candor will "kill" him is a self-fulfilling prophecy, for he cannot fully face his real self.

Phillip's heart attack differs from Sylvia's paralysis insofar as it is a disease with an ascertainable pathology. But the psychosomatic element in cardiovascular syndromes has long been acknowledged; all the textbooks on psychosomatic disorders include sections on the cardiovascular system.[10] The mechanism can be fully explained: stress, notably anger, raises blood pressure, and if the pressure remains elevated on account of continued, chronic stress, constriction of the arteries will result. This scenario clearly applies to Phillip. Unlike Sylvia's paralysis, his sickness cannot be deemed predominantly psychosomatic. Still, the burden of his long-standing guilty secret undoubtedly contributes to his collapse and death. In many respects he is sicker than his wife, for he has knowingly lived with his shame. He is also full of resentment and suspicion, believing that Sylvia is trying to destroy him (83). In these accusations against his wife, Phillip is trying to shift the guilt from himself onto her, without success, however; even though Dr. Hyman assures him that "it's not a trick" (76), he is unable to dislodge the anger.

As the curtain drops, Phillip lies in the throes of death, felled by a second heart attack. The word used to describe him as he falls back is, interestingly, "unconscious" (138). It refers primarily to his physical state, yet metaphorically it can also be read as denoting his incapacity to live with a conscious understanding of the pain he has inflicted on himself, on his wife, possibly even on his son. As a result of his programmatic concealment, his life had become one long falsehood which he cannot redeem. As he crumples to the floor, *his* legs now turned to butter, Sylvia "*struggles to balance herself on her legs and takes a faltering step toward her husband. . . . Astounded, charged with hope yet with a certain inward seeing, she looks down at her legs, only now aware that she has risen to her feet*" (138). Sylvia's legs regain their strength through her readiness to forgive, expressed in her cries, "Wait, wait. Phillip, Phillip!" (138), and through the "inward seeing" of consciously knowing, grasping, and coming to terms with what had happened in the course of her marriage. So she is able to break out of the loops of stress and repression that resulted in first her emotional and then her physical paralysis. While Phillip's confrontation of his past completes his disempowerment in death, hers brings her to the self-empowerment of taking possession of her examined life. The struggle for ascendancy in the Gellburg marriage is over. Sylvia, "buxom" and "capable," finally turns out to be the truly strong one, while Phillip is unmasked as an autocrat who merely feigned power.

This is the major instance of the reversals that characterize *Broken Glass*. Opening with Phillip's visit to Dr. Hyman's office to discuss Sylvia's illness, the play ends with her recovery and his death. The chiasmus is fully accomplished as he falls from his initial position of overbearing dictator in the household and she rises to find, first, words and, through them, self-affirmation. On the one hand, this structure of symmetries and antitheses is satisfying, particularly in the theater, making for a neat, well-constructed play. On the other hand, the play's design seems just too orderly. The contrast between the two couples, the tense, warring Gellburgs and the idyllically consonant Hymans (despite their differences in religion and background) seems overly simple.

Similarly, in keeping with this schema of reversals and symmetries, the ending of *Broken Glass* is excessively neat and somewhat contrived. Phillip's death, though well motivated, provides a very convenient conclusion to the problem by shortcircuiting it. Having regained her freedom and found out what she wants to do, Sylvia will in her widowhood likely return to business. With more women entering the workforce during World War II, this seems a reasonable hypothesis. Phillip's death on stage gives dramatic closure to the play, but what does this imply for Sylvia's conversion disorder? In the short run, her difficulties are over through removal of the major cause; but in the long run, has her capacity to understand herself and to deal with others changed sufficiently to avoid a repetition? Psychosomatic disorders tend to recur. If she were to remarry, would she prove to have learnt to relate differently to her husband? Much would depend on *his* personality and expectations. What is more, social conditions began to improve for women in World War II when they were granted a more active role in the war effort and consequently in public life. But the real question at the end of *Broken Glass* is this: what would have happened if Phillip had not succumbed to his second heart attack? Would Sylvia have regained use of her legs? Would the Gellburgs have been able to reconstruct their marriage on a healthier, more reciprocal basis? Could they have resumed sexual relations? Such changes would have denoted a genuine recovery on Sylvia's (and Phillip's) part. However, his death forecloses these possibilities.

Broken Glass offers a classic textbook example of a conversion disorder. Sylvia's paralysis is the linchpin to the play in its function as a startling pointer to the conflict that has for years remained latent and silent in the Gellburgs' marriage. From this perspective, it is the ideal text for the study of the portrayal of psychosomatic disorders in literature. Yet ultimately it is just too transparent. From Phillip's first appearance and his conversation with Dr. Hyman, despite his genuine concern for his wife, he becomes suspect as the source of Sylvia's distress because he is clearly such a devious and self-righteous person, who must make an objectionable husband. Miller is clever in inserting alternative, misleading clues to Sylvia's paralysis, notably her alarm at the events in Germany. This layering of explanations serves to heighten the suspense and hold the audience's attention until gradually, bit by bit, the true cause is uncovered.

In Sylvia's rising to her legs as the curtain drops, *Broken Glass* projects the potential for a positive outcome to her conversion disorder. Its role in Sylvia's life is as an idiom for the distress that had become intolerable. After a temporary decline into invalidism, Sylvia is helped through empathetic, supportive psychotherapy to reevaluate and consequently to reconstruct her life. So the play not only shows how the insidious accumulation of unresolved traumas can produce a psychosomatic disorder but also suggests that the removal of its ulterior causes can foster healing. But here again we come up against the tidy closure with Phillip's death, which is, paradoxically, not unconvincing but still too opportune. The prospect of a happy ending for Sylvia seems rather optimistic. So *Broken Glass* has a double face. On the one hand, it is a realistic, psychologically credible analysis of a conversion disorder; on the other hand, its schematic symmetries and its happy ending created by the combination of an exceptional family doctor and an expedient death turn it into something of a fairy-tale.[11]

CHAPTER NINE

Substance and Shadow

Brian O'Doherty, *The Strange Case of Mademoiselle P.* (1992)

For we know in part.
—*Corinthians* 13:9

"We are both substance and shadow, and it is the shadow that moves the substance" (7), the narrating voice asserts in the opening section of *The Strange Case of Mademoiselle P.* This phrase also applies to O'Doherty's novel as a whole. Its substance is the reconstruction of the historical case of the treatment of Marie-Therese von Paradies (1759–1824) by Dr. Franz Anton Mesmer (1734–1815) in Vienna in 1777.[1] Shadow is cast by the multiplicity of possible interpretations of the actual events and the consequent uncertainties in readers' minds. But it is precisely these ambivalences that make the novel so intriguing as they imaginatively capture the equivocations innate to psychosomatic disorders: are they substantive manifestations of a somatic disease or shadows of a psychological disturbance?

Marie-Therese was the daughter of Joseph von Paradies, private secretary to the Austro-Hungarian empress Maria-Theresa, after whom she was named. Born with perfect sight, she went blind overnight at age three on 9 December 1762, and remained so despite all the efforts of the medical faculty at the empress's behest on behalf of her godchild. She had been made to undergo a series of painful, gruesome, and disfiguring treatments, including leeches, bleeding, electric shocks, and a tight plaster cast on her head, all to no avail. But her blindness had not prevented her remarkable development in many respects. She had a pleasing personality, showed artistic ability, studied music under the great Viennese teacher, Leopold Kozeluch, and entertained the royal family. In recognition of her talent and as compensation for her disability, the empress awarded her a pension.

She was skilled at lace making too, and had altogether adapted very well to living with her blindness. Yet her parents still sought a cure, and therefore brought her to Mesmer on 20 January 1777, when she was eighteen years old, as a last resort. This is where the novel starts.

For Mesmer the arrival of a prominent patient in a pitiful condition and with an affliction so obdurate that it had defied Vienna's best doctors was the ideal opportunity to prove the efficacy of his theories and methods by effecting a spectacular cure. The Viennese medical world was at that time at best indifferent, or more frequently, antagonistic to Mesmer, although he had completed regular training, graduating in Vienna in 1766 with a dissertation on the influence of the planets on the human body, a topic unexceptional in the eighteenth century. Mesmer argued for a material cause of the planets' influence through what he called "universal fluid," in which all things are immersed as in a cosmic ocean; he maintained that this fluid determined not only gravitation but also magnetism, electricity, light, and heat. He had a tendency to grandiose speculation and was also suspected of association with secret societies. But after his marriage in 1768 to a wealthy widow of noble descent, Anna-Maria von Bosch, he settled to a largely conventional practice. Entertaining at their elegant home, the Mesmers took an active part in the city's high society and were informed patrons of the arts, especially music. Mesmer played the clavichord and the cello and was among the earliest champions of the glass harmonica, an older instrument then newly improved by Benjamin Franklin. He knew Mozart's father and hosted the first performance of the young Mozart's opera *Bastien and Bastienne* in the autumn of 1768.

The major turning-point in Mesmer's career occurred through his treatment of Franziska Oesterlin (known as "Franzl"), a relative of Mesmer's wife in her twenties. She suffered from a medley of ills: convulsions, spasms of vomiting, inflammation of the intestines, inability to urinate, toothache and earache, despondency, hallucinations, cataleptic trances, fainting spells, temporary blindness, feelings of suffocation, and attacks of paralysis. Franzl's diffuse symptoms foreshadow those of Anna O and of Emmy von N . . . in Breuer's and Freud's *Studies on Hysteria*. Mesmer recognized them as telltale signs of the syndrome then called hysteria. During 1773–74 he treated her successfully with magnets; she regained her health, married Mesmer's stepson, and led a normal life. However, when Mesmer sought to have his magnetic cure for nervous illnesses formally acknowledged by the medical faculty, his claims were rejected. From this time on Mesmer had a dubious reputation. His cure of Franzl earned him some patients but also the lasting distrust and hostility of the medical establishment. This then is the historical context for *The Strange Case of Mademoiselle P.* Both the broad contours of Mesmer's career and details such as the names of the physicians who were Mesmer's enemies correspond to known facts.

The tensions in the medical field are closely connected to those at the empress's court, where the doctors vied for patients and, even more, for favors. The rivalries, jealousies, gossip, jostling for position, and malice are vividly evoked, especially in the fourth section of the novel, which centers on Joseph von Paradies. Large issues such as the disagreements on foreign policy between the empress and her son serve not merely as a backdrop to the central drama of the treatment of Marie-Therese, but also suggest the archetypal pervasiveness of intergenerational conflicts. This is one of the ways in which the social dimension is more immediately relevant to the plot than may at first be apparent.

The deviousness customary in behavior at court is a reiterated theme. Courtiers do not speak their minds openly for fear of offending an influential person or assuming a position that may prove unpropitious. Joseph von Paradies complains about the role imposed on him as intermediary between the empress and her son: "I was constantly on the go between her and her son, the Emperor, rephrasing one of her comments in a diplomatic way and similarly translating his reply. Why they didn't talk to each other directly is a mystery to me" (80). His lament is ironic, for Joseph knows perfectly well that no one talks directly at court. Hypocrisy is the norm, the mask the public visage. Spies and assassins are said to go about "wearing the mask of decent folk" (98), and even at concerts, the courtiers' "attention is a mask for wandering thoughts, . . . since simulating attention is the main trade" (17). While forthright communication is spurned as dangerous, gossip and slander circulate readily in "this porous court" (108). The habit of dissimulation, intrinsic to the court, is a determining factor in the creation of the shadows in this novel. The court hangs like a shadow over the entire action as a major "intermediate variable."[2] Where deviousness is the rule, nothing can be accepted at face value. Utterances, conduct, and motivation are all subject to unremitting suspicion.

The mistrust of Mesmer by the physicians allied with the court is one instance of this ubiquitously poisonous atmosphere. The doctors charged with examining Marie-Therese's eyes to verify Mesmer's claim to improvement are all described as engaged in posturing. Dr. Barth adopts a grave, semilistening pose; Dr. Ost has perfected his façade, and Dr. Ingenhousz's face says "doctor" so loudly that "when I heard children cry in the back of the house as I was leaving, my fancy was that he took off his face when he returned to these quarters to beget them" (110). This image of donning and shedding a public face is a graphic way of conveying the pervasiveness of simulation. Deceit colors even the scientific activities under the auspices of the court. As all the court physicians had failed to cure Marie-Therese, Mesmer realizes that his success would only "inflame" (7) the opposition to him still further. Mesmer himself is, therefore, from the outset in two minds, wanting very much to cure the girl, but at the same time afraid of retribution.

Mesmer's hesitations reveal the web of dependency at court as an intricate system built on the reciprocal exchange of favors. Joseph von Paradies's life is one long pursuit of favors, indicated by little gestures as well as by promises. He fawns and grovels before anyone thought to wield power: "I recognized him as the Dr. Ost who was made court physician last year. So I suddenly became all ears and showed him every good manner. I had thought he was someone's relative looking for a favor at court—which I am pleased to grant if it is in my power, depending, of course, on their ability to return it later" (130–31). To Mesmer, Joseph von Paradies seems "one of those careful men one finds around court, who while watching the weather vane maintains a distance which passes for dignity and is often mistaken for wisdom" (6). Uncertainty about a person's status causes Joseph confusion: "'To what end is your visit, sir?' . . . I knew nothing of this man's connections and could not inflect my responses to his interests" (135). The inauthenticity that is the hallmark of the court makes it extremely difficult to distinguish between substance and shadow. To do so is the aim of both the characters and of readers.

The difficulty of achieving this aim is vastly compounded for readers by this short novel's narrative disposition. Each of its five sections is a first-person narration, emanating from three different voices. In the first, second, and fifth chapters, it is Mesmer's voice; in the third, Marie-Therese's; and in the fourth, her father's. Of the four main characters in the novel, only the mother remains voiceless and her thoughts opaque, except insofar as they can be deduced from the others' accounts. The first four sections are contemporaneous, dealing with the time of Marie-Therese's treatment by Mesmer and its immediate aftermath. By contrast, the fifth, Mesmer's retrospective reflections on the events of 1777, dates from 1814, the year before his death. Of increasing length and complexity, the chapters evolve from the predominantly reportorial to the largely speculative. So the narrative itself moves from substance to shadow.

The shadowiness is most evident in the final chapter. At age eighty, Mesmer is in a reminiscent mood as he recalls his past, especially the attempted cure of Marie-Therese. Mimicking the drift of his consciousness, the format is associative and rambling as current experiences meld with dreams and memories. The landscape "is topsy-turvy," for thoughts "play leapfrog and hide" (164) in his mind. In a drawer he finds an old manuscript, "a little graveyard of the past" (200), written shortly after the events of 1777, and from it he retrieves the passages concerning Marie-Therese. The intercalation of materials from an old, recently discovered manuscript is a common enough literary device; it further distances the action from readers through the intervention of another frame, and so heightens the mystery. For Mesmer the effect is "a sense of double displacement from both my present and my past, as if a third party were reading and listening to my earlier self speaking in the present tense of a present long perished" (202). That "sense of a double displacement" is experienced by readers too as they try to attain clarity. In this endeavor, their aim coincides with Mesmer's for the purpose of his ruminations about his past is to disentangle the rumors that have come to surround his treatment of Marie-Therese from the facts as he remembers them. But "rumor has certified fiction as fact" (159). Was he, for instance, present in the audience at the concert she gave, as a *blind* pianist, in Paris in 1784? Mesmer maintains that he never saw her again after he left Vienna in 1778, but he was in Paris in 1784, so a meeting might have taken place.[3] Certain at first that he had not been there, "over the years, the most peculiar thing has happened. I find myself beginning to concur with those witnesses who vouch for my presence" (160). At question is not so much the meeting itself as the nature of Mesmer's relationship to Marie-Therese. A slippage occurs in Mesmer's own consciousness, so that he finds himself "in two minds these days, or, perhaps more truly, between two minds" (153). His history "divides into two histories in which the real events are banal and forgotten and the fictional ones thoroughly convincing to the world at large, and even, in moments of attention, to myself" (162).

Once "doubt has entered the chambers of my own mind and heart" (199), shadow tends to become substance. In his manuscript Mesmer had written of seeing "a proven truth redirected, little by little, into an area of uncertainty and conjecture" (219); his phrase refers to Marie-Therese's cure, but it summarizes too what happens to him in the course of his reminiscing. Ruefully, he concludes, that he has "watched while error assumed the face of truth and, so masked, drew to it the approval of those who reject the genuine in favor of a substitute" (222). The words "masked" and the rejection of "the genuine in favor of the substitute" link the realm of private life with the behavior at court. In the world created in *The Strange Case of Mademoiselle P.* there are only "versions" (52) of the story, subjectively perceived, shaped by prejudices and preconceptions, distorted in part subconsciously and in part to advance personal agendas. Through its clever design, the novel provides variants, all of which hover in a precarious perspectivism between substance and shadow. Each narrating voice presents his or her own view, and even these may moderate, as Mesmer's successive accounts show; none can be accepted as reliable; final truth is beyond reach within this novel.

"And who can better tell truth from falsehood than I?" asks Marie-Therese. "I, who is the darkness at their center" (52). The darkness of her blindness here takes on a metaphorical dimension. As in *Broken Glass,* the physical manifestation of the psychosomatic disorder is plainly evident. Also as in *Broken Glass,* its psychosocial origins are complicated, rooted in the two intersecting circles of the public and the private context. The court intrigues in *The Strange Case of Mademoiselle P.* correspond as outer influences to Crystal Night in Miller's play. The private realm in both instances hinges on family dynamics. However, the two works differ in their outcome. While *Broken Glass* offers both a resolution and an explanation of Sylvia's paralysis, *The Strange Case of Mademoiselle P.* remains just that: strange, resistant to definitive resolution on either the physical or the psychosocial plane. Unlike Sylvia, Marie-Therese is, despite her contention, unable to tell truth from falsehood any better than the other figures in this challenging novel.

While all the characters are enigmatic, none are more so than Marie-Therese's parents. They remain largely shadows in the text; nevertheless, they come to assume a distinctive substance in readers' minds. This holds particularly true for Marie-Therese's mother, who comes across from the very first sentences onward as a domineering personality: "She [Marie-Therese] said nothing, but drifted towards me. Her mother, who had arranged this meeting, was voluble, dividing her discourse between respectful address to me and sharp cautions to her daughter" (3). As a young, unmarried woman in the eighteenth century, Marie-Therese would naturally still be under her parents' tutelage. In the novel's opening section we see both her and her mother exclusively through Mesmer's eyes. He realizes at once that Marie-Therese has been conditioned to obedience and submissiveness; her facial expression is "patient, though at this time a little anxious" (4), and, not unexpectedly, he finds her "somewhat passive, but that passivity, it seemed to me, was a result of a highly developed patience" (12). The image of the mother, however, is decidedly negative. She weeps inordinately, wails and whines, sobs exaggeratedly, and starts to "babble in a way that seemed to me to have much precedent" (4). The suggestion that she is putting on a routine performance to elicit sympathy seems to be confirmed by her self-pitying effusiveness: "[W]hat have we done to deserve such torment—our only child" (5). She has no sensitivity whatsoever to her daughter's plight. She appears to be so villainous as to prompt readers much rather to ask what it is that the parents had done to their only child to trigger so extreme a reaction as a conversion blindness at age three.

This initial encounter with Marie-Therese's mother gives Mesmer his "first inkling that it would be necessary to separate the child from the mother" (5). His fundamental proviso for undertaking any treatment, to which her parents accede with reluctance, is that she "should live in my clinic, away from the everyday influence of her mother" (10). This proviso is allegedly motivated by the need for the patient's full attention, but Mesmer wonders how much her parents had contributed to her condition" (10). The mother's emotional vehemence, self-centeredness, and posses-siveness arouse the suspicion of parental implication in the etiology of Marie-Therese's blindness. Mesmer's examination of her eyes quickly convinces him of the absence of any pathology: "The pupils responded to light. The eyes were alive, but separated from the light by a darkness of the mind" (10). As soon as he has established that the deficit is psychosomatic, not physical, Mesmer is willing to attempt a cure. But his efforts to find out anything about the onset of the blindness meet with a complete blank: "Why a three-year-old child should suddenly become blind was mysterious, and mysterious to her mother, who assigned the responsibility to a Godly whim" (11). The circumstances surrounding the onset of Marie-Therese's disorder are never brought to light; they remain central unexplained shadows in this novel, to be grasped only by readers' constructive conjectures.

The suspicion of the parents' involvement in the blindness is supported by the change in Marie-Therese when she is removed from their orbit: "she flourished like a spring flower," Mesmer notes (12). He observes too that her mother's daily visits are "not pleasant" to her, although "she wore a pleasing smile" (12). In addition to patience and submissiveness, Marie-Therese has already learnt something of the masking necessary in her environment. During her mother's daily and her father's twice-weekly visits, she "was both present and far away" (12) as if she had acquired the habit of seeming to be present while inwardly practicing a self-protective absence. The phrase "present and far away" is a fitting description of the effect of her blindness; it is a way of dealing with a disagreeable present by distancing or abstracting herself. These many small hints early on in *The Strange Case of Mademoiselle P.* insinuate the idea forming in Mesmer's mind that the parents are a decisive factor in Marie-Therese's disorder. Her conversation provides the alert Mesmer with another clue, for it "flowed easily except when I discussed her family life or her illness. The rhythmic nodding of her body then became more exaggerated and rapid, and the smile became an anguished grin, like the tragic mask in the theater" (13). Debarred by the conventions of her society from expressing feelings openly, Marie-Therese speaks instead through her body.

The scenario of the strife within this family coalesces cumulatively from a series of episodes recorded from various angles. In the opening two chapters, narrated by Mesmer, he follows his conviction of the parents' deleterious impact on Marie-Therese by doing his utmost to keep them away from her. In the third section, in which Marie-Therese gives her version, there is no overt criticism, partly out of ingrained filial obligations, and partly out of fear of their retribution. In this network of "favors," a daughter must stay in her parents' favor. However, she is acutely aware of the shrill disagreements between her mother and father as she overhears their quarrels: "My father's tones did not diminish, but drew my mother's whispers to almost the same volume—if you can imagine a whispered shout—which seemed to increase my father's distemper. The sounds of their voices confused me. When I closed my eyes, their voices issued from the corner of the room where their persons were located. But when I opened my eyes, they seemed to issue every which way, first from one place and then another, so that it seemed to me a company of mothers and fathers arguing like furies" (64). This is the strongest language ever to come from the otherwise gentle Marie-Therese; it testifies to the deep emotional disturbance she suffers in this atmosphere of antagonisms. What is more, she has learnt that by closing her eyes she is able to confine the querulous voices to the corner of the room her parents occupy, whereas when she opens her eyes she feels as if surrounded by "a company of . . . furies." Closing off her sight permanently is thus a way of insulating herself. In the only reference to her childhood, she recalls that from her earliest days her father "had the ability to signify his disapproval with a silence that invaded my darkness like a fog. My mother now joined him frequently, and they resumed their arguments, adding to my troubles" (74). As she begins to regain some sight under Mesmer's care and is thus on the road to emancipation from her parents' domination, their censure of her grows ever more strident.

The strife escalates into actual physical violence when her parents come forcibly to remove her from Mesmer's clinic. Marie-Therese remembers weeping and crying as her father scuttles in, brandishing a sword: "My mother shrieked at me, as she had done many times when I was a child, rushed at me, half-embraced me, then flung me from her against the wall, which seemed to rise to strike me" (76). This melee marks the moment when Marie-Therese suddenly and irrevocably relapses into blindness. Since she explicitly aligns this incident with many similar ones in her childhood, it seems likely that some such aggression had contributed to precipitating her initial withdrawal into blindness. Naturally, her parents would deny any knowledge of causes. But the father's narrative contains further glimpses of the abusiveness habitual in this family. He recounts that on her return home, Marie-Therese weeps "for no cause but her own sense of misery, which irritated her mother out of her wits, so that she began to scold and beat her, which provoked me greatly. It is not true that I have treated my wife in like fashion, as you may have heard from those vile fellows at court, who heard it from their wives, to whom my wife exaggerates everything" (83). In this realm of hypocrisy, Joseph von Paradies's point-blank denial stimulates the conjecture of precisely the opposite, namely that he *has* treated his wife in like fashion. He is greatly troubled not by the abuse itself but by the fact that word of his viciousness has spread through court gossip, damaging his image. He shows more concern for his reputation than for the crass behavior in his household. The shadow takes precedence over the substance in private within the home as well as in public at court.

The dynamics of this sick family triangle are clearly articulated by Mesmer in his concluding reflections: "Of course she was blind, since the matter was in her organ's function, not its structure, and that function was occluded by her circumstances, if we can call her parents 'circumstances'" (159). He accuses her father point-blank: "You bully the sight out of her" (75).

Where does Marie-Therese stand in this struggle between her parents and her healer? Does her physical blindness bestow on her the capacity for deeper insight because she is not distracted by surface appearances? Can she "tell truth from falsehood"?

The first impression is of her innocence. Mesmer and all his household find her "a person of extraordinary sweetness" (12). She rapidly responds to their genuine kindness, taking to Mesmer's wife as a surrogate mother. Yet she is not quite as disingenuous as she initially appears. In compensation for her lack of sight, she has heightened aural acuity, so that as she hears "the conflicting voices argue my fate and my future," she is aware of how "they betray their thoughts by the way their words are spoken" (52). Does this imply that she can hear in her parents' discourse their manipulativeness? While she hints at this possibility, she never puts it into words. Her youth, gender, and guilelessness prevent her from having the detachment or overview of the total situation to comprehend the duplicitous game being played with her. The model of her docile subjection is enacted as she lets her father guide her to the piano and prompt her performance. This ritual carries a metaphorical meaning in showing Marie-Therese being directed like a puppet on a string controlled by her father.

But if she is disempowered by her blindness, she is also curiously empowered by it. Her skill in lace making astonishes Mesmer and, even more so, the assurance of her piano playing. She evokes not mere sympathy for a disabled person but the admiration and amazement of the empress and her courtiers for her accomplishments. A poised young woman, she projects "a feminine presence" (20). While her blindness injects a certain pathos into her existence, she seems to have made up for her deficit by developing talents dependent on touch and hearing. She has instinctively found reparations for what she cannot do.

The retrieval of her sight surprisingly brings more problems than rewards. O'Doherty's evocation of the process of returning sight is highly imaginative, as he traces Marie-Therese's confusion at her first glimpse of a human face, her perplexity at understanding perspective and distance, and especially her difficulties in connecting various common objects to their names without the intermediacy of touch. The conventions of language are an enormous mystery and challenge to her. The sighted state is full of shocks to Marie-Therese, who still remains "in the infancy of her sight" (75) when her parents withdraw her from Mesmer's care before she has had the time to make the necessary adjustments.

Through seeing, Marie-Therese acquires some important capacities previously beyond her ken. Contact with the natural world of flowers and dogs is the earliest among her new pleasures. She is utterly captivated by the night sky with its contrast between darkness and light and its beautiful stars. Her deepest empowerment derives from her discovery of her budding sexuality. O'Doherty takes the liberty of slightly amending historical happenings by making the young Mozart a frequent visitor to Mesmer's house during Marie-Therese's stay. She had probably met Mozart earlier, and certainly did so later, in Salzburg in 1783, when he wrote the B-flat concerto (K. 456) for her. However, O'Doherty concedes in a postscript that "it is unlikely that Mlle. Paradies enountered Mozart during her treatment with Dr. Mesmer" (229). This deliberate revision of historical fact fulfills a cardinal purpose in the novel: that of revealing the unfolding of Marie-Therese's adult feelings. At first, the duets she plays with Mozart "are the greatest joy to me" (69), but soon superimposed on this is the thrill of his physical closeness: "Sitting side by side on the long stool, I am aware with Wolfgang of things that perhaps he is not. Sometimes, reaching over to the treble, his arm brushes against my bosom in a way that adds a note of pleasure to the notes that are flocking around us. I think of this more than I should, and must confess that at times I have not been disinclined to lean my bosom to where his arm must brush it" (70). Like Sylvia in *Broken Glass,* Marie-Therese is able to recognize the potency of her sexual drive and to take possession of her feelings.

Still, Marie-Therese experiences sight as "more a terror than a blessing" (37). Her mental state, Mesmer observes, "began to be ruffled," and she seems to have "unlearned the room" (28), falling over the few pieces of furniture more frequently than in her unsighted somnambulism. Her physical and psychological equilibrium is disturbed. Most distressing to her is her inability to read musical notes. Her fingers at the piano, formerly a tool of empowerment, are here a synecdoche for her entire persona in signifying her paradoxical *loss* of independence in her new sighted state. Since Mozart witnesses her "hesitation and distress" (72), her ineptitude, indeed her failure through her production of "poor music" (72) is a humiliation to her. Vision comes to seem "a doubtful blessing" (62).

Marie-Therese's position is complicated by her extraordinary adaptation to her blindness during the previous fifteen years. In the frustrations of trying to learn the basic task of eating, for instance, Mesmer notes that: "Again and again, when in such difficulty, she would close her eyes, returning to that secure darkness in which she had negotiated fifteen years of her life so successfully" (33). Blindness denotes security to Marie-Therese. It enables her symbolically as well as literally to shut out the world and to live in her self-created realm of musical accord. Above all, her blindness is a means at least partially to shut out her parents. However, she does not realize, as Mesmer does, the extent to which she "had become a pawn in a game involving the court, the medical profession, [his] household" (213). He sees her "struggles against her affliction like those of a fly in a web" (213). She is a pawn to her parents' greed and ambition; it is in their interest to keep her as a sightless wonder so as to remain assured of the pension awarded to her by the empress.

Is Marie-Therese unconsciously complicit in their maneuvers because the apparent disempowerment of the sick role grants her a more significant empowerment in other respects? This is one of the most troubling questions at the heart of *The Strange Case of Mademoiselle P.* She has no choice about returning to the parental home. But what is the implicit message as she speaks at that point through her body by reverting to blindness? She downplays her physical handicap to concentrate more on the emotional aspects: "I do not deny my infirmity, which I never think of as my dead eyes, but as that infection of the emotions I catch from others, especially those near to me" (54). With her hypersensitivity to the undertones of speech, she surely picks up on her parents' inability to accept her regained sight. She comments that "they must have felt me replaced by another person" (63), as if she were a sinister changeling. And she could not have avoided registering her father's vehement outburst: "The girl is now a shadow of herself. Look at her. She cannot play. She understands nothing. She has become a child" (74). Does she want to go back to being the good child rather than the disappointing one? On the one hand, she expresses her sense of guilt and responsibility toward her parents for the problems caused by her disability: "When my parents fell into a mood, I always presumed that I was the cause, and so had a habit of feeling guilty. I always felt my dead eyes were a burden to them" (62–63). On the other hand, she may have heard them speak of their fear of losing her pension, and so realize that she is of greater benefit to them sightless. Which is the shadow, and which the substance? It is conceivable that Marie-Therese can indeed tell truth from falsehood, but if so, she is unable to act on her insight.

Mesmer is the one who makes the most concerted effort to tell truth from falsehood, substance from shadow, as he seeks in the closing chapter to sort out the real nature of his relationship to Marie-Therese and to sift rumor from fact. In so doing, he uncovers the unsettled and unsettling disparity between conscious and subconscious motivations.

Mesmer's introspection is prompted by a dream that radically subverts his self-image:

> [I]n my dream, she posed before me, drifting through the darkened room, urgently followed by my desire, in a way totally at variance with the facts. For I never desired her. I was to her a father, and she to me a child by proxy. In my dream, in that distant darkness, I stroked her body to coax the magnetic fluids to circulate to her afflicted eyes, gathering them from limbs and body to bring light to her eyes— . . . I never disrobed her. I simply reached under her costume, with my own eyes closed, to share her condition, and there stroked gently as was demanded by my therapy. But in my unwanted dream, thirty years later, her bare thighs glimmered in the twilight while I stroked them from inside the knee to the vicinity of her sex, before which, as God is my judge and my wife is my witness, I stopped short. This dream has tortured me, for it is not consistent with my memory, nor with my opinion of myself, and thus has pained me greatly. (143–44)

Which is the substance, which the shadow? What offers the more accurate account: Mesmer's memory or his dream?

Nor is this dream an isolated occurence. A second dream, too, leaves Mesmer "much disturbed" (167). This time, as he seems to "glide down a corridor, unconscious of [his] motion and with no feeling of unease or dread," he comes upon a young woman whose hands are flying over a piano keyboard as she plays the *Lied der Blindheit*, song on blindness, which Marie-Therese had composed and which had greatly moved him. Then as

> these thoughts occupied me in my dream, my hands, to
> my horror, slipped from her shoulders to her bosom. The
> pianist raised her hands from the keyboard, fingers spread
> wide; she stretched her head directly back so that I saw it
> upside-down from above. Marie-Therese's expression was
> one of utter terror, the eyes again showing nothing but the
> whites, as if she were trying to look at me through her own
> skull and substance. The shock was so intense that I woke
> up with my heart beating in a flutter of irregularities.
> (168–69)

The overt sexual content of these dreams causes Mesmer such profound agitation in part because they revive charges that had been made against him, not only in regard to Marie-Therese but to other women patients as well. Now the dreams are raising the shadow of those same accusations: "[I]n the light of day I refuted the charges. This had never happened. But a suspicion remained" (170). "I never touched her profanely," he insists in his waking state. Yet in a third dream he visualizes her as standing before him "entirely naked, her body still half childish with young breasts and scanty sex" (195). Reminding himself "in a great convulsion of effort" of his "fatherly role," he "embraced her reassuringly" (196). But this pure vision is overtaken by another one: "[I]n the darkness, her body filled out, her arms around me became knowing and suggestive. Their caresses appealed to something dark in my being. In an animal darkness, a violent passion seized me of an order unknown to me in my prime" (196). Awaking, he perceives himself, eighty years old, sitting on the side of his bed, "lusting after a young girl of eighteen"—by then herself forty-five.

In these dreams, as "the body grumbles its way into consciousness" (151), Mesmer's unconscious is forcing him to confront highly unpalatable possibilities. He emphatically protests his recoil from these scenarios over and again; the first dream is "unwanted" and "inconsistent with my memory," while the acts in the second are "to my horror." He attributes the dreams to his "body" because he believes them, like psychosomatic disorders, to emanate from a disturbance of the distribution "in the magnetic fluid" (170) that affects the physical system. Do his dreams express the profane desire for her that he vociferously denies in the waking state? However insistently he rejects the idea, "a doubt had been placed in my mind, which, no matter how I rehearse my past, I cannot cast out" (170). Where, he asks, "does this grotesque revision of my history come from? Why should my mind betray me in this fashion?" (145).

Mesmer can barely countenance that it may be his conscious memory, not his mind, that is betraying him. The "grotesque revision" of his history may be a manifestation of wishes he had repressed; the subconscious desires then surface in the dreams. Whether he had actually violated Marie-Therese or not is beside the point. The wish had been there, and thirty-seven years later it comes back literally to haunt his dreams. No more than Marie-Therese can Mesmer tell truth from falsehood. He applies the adjective "blind" (151) to himself, and, continuing the imagery of sight, infers of his memory that "my nose is too close to the window to see what is on the glass" (163).

That phrase is apposite to readers of *The Strange Case Mademoiselle P.* We, too, are so close to the window that it is hard to see exactly what is on the glass. This dilemma results from the narrative disposition as a sequence of first-person accounts that mostly complement but at times contradict each other, creating ambiguities and uncertainties. Yet we have to attempt to see through the glass to construct the story, even if we cannot with final assurance tell truth from falsehood.

We are impeded in so doing by the secrecy encoded in the novel. All the main protagonists keep secrets from themselves as well as from each other. This resistance to possible, unpalatable truths by the conscious mind becomes most apparent in Mesmer's dreams, which make him face a story very different from that he has cherished, but it occurs also in the other characters.

With Marie-Therese the situation is complex. Out of filial loyalty and constraint by conventions, she seeks to conceal and suppress what may be her true—but inadmissible—feelings for her parents. Right at the outset Mesmer notes that "there is much that is hidden about her" (20). Though at first she manages to produce the expected (rigid) smile at her mother's unpleasant visits, her behavior changes as her cure progresses. Still speaking primarily through her body, she begins to shake at her mother's annoyance "at what she thought my stupidity" (56). As she is released from her blindness and from her emotional enthralment to her parents, she learns to be more open; she can speak in words rather than through her body. She refuses to see her mother for several days; this refusal coincides with the time when she is discovering her own body in the joyful consonance of the duets with Mozart. From then on she develops "a distaste for her mother," her father reports, and shows "a reluctance to discuss her feelings with me" (93). In his demand for her return home, he complains among other things of "her most undaughterly feelings for her parents" (131). Marie-Therese seems to "know in part," as it is put in *Corinthians,* and to acknowledge in part the true feelings behind the crumbling façade. To what extent does she attain self-awareness, or does she continue to block out what she cannot face? Self-assertive rebellion was not an option for an eighteen-year-old girl of good family in the eighteenth century. Once she is forced home, she falls back into the role society imposes on her—and into the sole expression of her emotions available to her, through her body, negatively in her blindness, and positively in her fingers at the piano.

Of the mother we know least at first hand, because she herself has no narrative, so that we have to judge her from others' accounts. The distortions inherent in the subjectivity of first-person narration are therefore compounded by the intervention of a mediating perception. To Mesmer certainly and increasingly to Marie-Therese she appears as acrimonious and malevolent. Of her abuse of her daughter there can be no doubt. Dr. Ost, the court physician, to whom the father appeals for help in securing Marie-Therese's return home, asks without circumlocution: "[I]s it true . . . that your wife on occasion has abused the girl?" (132). The father's reply is characteristically evasive in its reference to "domestic griefs" and to the "great strain" that has adversely affected his wife's health (133). This answer is tantamount to a veiled admission of the accusation. If Joseph von Paradies is protective of his wife, it is because she is in collusion with him.

The father is the most puzzling character since his experience of masking at court has made him a master of dissimulation. It is he, Marie-Therese recalls, who had "from my earliest years . . . urged me to the harpsichord, demanding long hours of practice" (58). She is relieved that Mesmer keeps him at a distance, but he eavesdrops on her playing and is angered at her confusion and loss of mastery as her sight returns. *The Strange Case of Mademoiselle P.* invites us to jump to the conclusion that he is motivated above all by financial considerations, that is, the possible forfeiture of Marie-Therese's pension if she is no longer handicapped.

But another scenario is also insinuated, one that connects the father's tyranny to the secret trigger to his daughter's blindness. Not satisfied with the mother's postulate that it was due to "a Godly whim," Mesmer speculates: "Did some awful sight present itself that left her mind no option but to eclipse it?" (11). That awful sight might have been a glimpse of her father as he raped her. This hypothesis is supported by Mesmer's observation that the father is "over-fond" of his daughter, and his intuition that he had "some monstrous thoughts" in his mind (197). Even more telling is

Marie-Therese's extreme revulsion, in Mesmer's second dream, at any sexual approach, which suggests a degree of dread far beyond normal virginal apprehensiveness: "Marie-Therese's expression was one of utter terror, the eyes again showing nothing but the whites, as if she were trying to look at me through her own skull and substance" (169). Here the disfigurement of the eyes is linked to the terror of a sexual advance by an older man. Her reaction takes on added significance in light of the fatherly role Mesmer had assumed toward her, so that he becomes associated in her mind with her childhood abuser. His dream shows her recuperating the memory of a previous rape perpetrated on her. She tries to "look through her own skull and substance" in order to banish that substance, even at the cost of living in shadow. In this reading, her blindness denotes the avoidance conversion of an experience of incest. And the mother, with at least partial knowledge of what had happened, is covering up to protect her husband's and the family's reputation. Her repeated discharge of inordinate rage reiterates her outrage at the original violence, that is, she is outing her rage. She, too, not coincidentally, is subject to a conversion disorder in her nervous ill health, for which she has consulted several physicians.

This interpretation of the latent plot of *The Strange Case of Mademoiselle P.* allows for a deeper understanding of the twisted relationships among the characters. The parents are bound together, like Phillip and Sylvia in *Broken Glass,* by a communal dark secret. Marie-Therese is only partially privy to that secret; she does not want to know or to *see* it. Mesmer, inevitably, is the father's antagonist. In aiming to open Marie-Therese's eyes literally on the physical level, he does so figuratively also to her parents' malignity and violation of her. Mesmer becomes a surrogate good father, who is subsequently unmasked in his desire for her as a rival to, and a repetition of, her own bad father. As both men strive to assert their power over her mind, they desire as well to possess her body. Terrified at witnessing these assaults, Marie-Therese averts her gaze and takes flight into blindness.

These conflicts are largely veiled in secrecy in the semi-consciousness of the characters and in the penumbra of the text. They are shadows rather than substances. The motif of blindness pervades the novel, and not only in regard to Marie-Therese. The court doctors who come to examine her improvement are impervious to the difficulties involved in the recovery of sight, notably the linguistic problem of attaching names to objects previously identified only by touch. They are, to some extent deliberately, blind to her progress because they are unwilling to concede Mesmer's success. Mesmer's verdict is that they suffer from "an inner blindness so profound that it darkens the name of science" (178). Likewise, Joseph von Paradies reproaches himself for his failure to see what he deems the true state of affairs: "It burst on me suddenly, . . . that the eyes that had been blinded were not my daughter's but my own. For with all the talk of improvement, with those trivial little litanies of progress . . . I had neglected the evidence of my eyes" (103). That evidence is supposed to enable him to tell truth from falsehood, but his interpretation of what he sees misleads him; Marie-Therese *is* improving, and he does not see, or *wish* to see that her confusion is an integral part of the process. The ambivalences of looking and seeing are hinted too in "that game of glances" constantly played at court where the meeting of eyes denotes a connection, whereas "the impact of a stare is almost like a slap" (25).[4] Had a glimpse of her father's stare as he raped her been the metaphoric "slap" that induced Marie-Therese's blindness? Nor is Mesmer exempt from the affliction of not seeing clearly. As he struggles to distinguish truth from falsehood in the dreams that assail him in old age, he feels at times "almost blinded" (195). In the literal darkness of the night, he is torn between his public, daylight self-perception as a benign healer and the recognition of "something dark in my being" (196). Like Marie-Therese, and like her parents, he has repressed images discomfiting to him.

Not seeing is partnered by not voicing. The text yields its secrets as reluctantly as do the characters. Decisive matters are not uttered but enacted, as in psychosomatic disorders. Communication between Marie-Therese and her parents is one-way, as they give orders and she obeys in silence. Only in the middle section of the novel, during her treatment by Mesmer, is she granted voice in her narrative. As her sight returns, so does her capacity for speech; conversely, after her relapse into blindness, she is not heard again. The parents, Mesmer notes, are not open to words: "Yesterday the father listened without listening, as indeed the mother did today" (8). By contrast, Marie-Therese is extremely receptive to voices and to their implications in their undertones.

In the complicated web of blindness and seeing, silence and shouting in *The Strange Case of Mademoiselle P.*, the distinction between truth and falsehood, substance and shadow remains to the very end elusive. Exactly how much conscious knowledge do the characters have of their actions, let alone their motivations? Was there some mysterious compatibility, some reciprocal response between Mesmer and Marie-Therese? He ponders that "there was something in her nature that spoke to some aspect of mine, as if we shared a secret, transmitted through a vibration of the magnetic fluid" (158). That eighteenth-century reference to magnetic fluid can readily be translated into modern terms of the transference and countertransference between patient and therapist. Or was it, as Mesmer's dreams suggest, primarily sexual in nature, at least on his side? If so, to what extent did Marie-Therese sense this feeling emanating from him? She is, indeed, as she claims, "the darkness at [the] center" (52) of this intriguing novel.

If Marie-Therese and Mesmer form the substance of *The Strange Case of Mademoiselle P.,* the shadow hanging over the entire work is that of Freud. The family romance as family tale of horror is a reiteration of the scenario that emerges from many of his famous cases, most notably Dora, but also Emmy von N . . . , Katharina, Elisabeth von R . . . , and Cäcilie, all in *Studies on Hysteria.* Like Marie-Therese, these women are injured and victimized in the strife that Freud uncovers in the depths of outwardly respectable families. Even though Freud jettisoned the seduction theory, he upheld his conviction that partially forgotten, partially repressed memories of early traumas are at the root of many later psychological disturbances. The possibility that Marie-Therese's conversion blindness is a response to rape by her father is certainly in keeping with Freudian beliefs. Still more obviously Freudian are Mesmer's "unwanted" (144) dreams, which force onto him the intense sexuality beneath his apparently fatherly stance toward his patient. The dictum attributed to Mesmer: "The mind itself is a shadow that inhabits our substance in elusive and contradictory ways" (7) anticipates the entire basis of psychoanalysis in which, as Theodor Reik so elegantly put it in *Listening with the Third Ear,* "Hard facts become shadows, and elusive shadows become facts."

A Freudian interpretation of *The Strange Case of Mademoiselle P.* is, from a strictly historical perspective, an anachronism. Mesmer has been cast as a forerunner of Freud in his use of suggestion and autosuggestion as therapeutic agencies,[5] but he did not have Freud's systematic understanding of the role of the unconscious. O'Doherty is in fact careful not to modernize Mesmer. Repeatedly throughout the novel mention is made of his beliefs in the harmonies between mind, body, and planets, and especially in "the invisible fluids that ebb and flow within each of our bodies" (11). In his treatment of Marie-Therese he spends hours, she recounts, "massaging [her] temples and forehead, to settle the disturbed fluids that had caught up [her] eyes in their agitation" (76). The eighteenth-century context is categorically evoked too by the multiple references to events and actual personages of the period, by the introduction of words with an archaic ring such as "distemper," "garbed," and "mantel," and by the projection of certain expectations of behavior, for instance between parents and a near-adult daughter. But this pronounced awareness of the eighteenth-century setting does not prevent readers from *also* interpreting from a twentieth-century angle, especially as the period environment functions almost as a decorative element that does not impinge on the timeless, archetypal nature of either the family conflict or of the sexually charged atmosphere. Thus in a further instance of the dualism of substance and shadow, space opens up for a dyadic reading of the novel. Mesmerian views represent a mask for the Freudian psychology underlying the plot.

This dualism is articulated when Marie-Therese compares herself to "a person with two languages (I have French in addition to my native German), one which put the world into reasonable order, the other which bore no relation to the world at all" (62). As readers, we also have two languages: one that constructs the overt text in eighteenth-century Mesmerian terms, and the other that probes its covert level in a Freudian interpretation. But ultimately the alternative is not between one or the other, between truth and falsehood, substance and shadow, for the two merge imperceptibly into a set of possibilities. Marie-Therese's blindness is the ideal symbol for these ambiguities adumbrated by O'Doherty with singular virtuosity. For a psychosomatic blindness is at once a real and a false blindness, a substantive and a shadowy disorder. It is, therefore, not only the subject but also the central metaphoric carrier of meaning in *The Strange Case of Mademoiselle P.*

CHAPTER TEN

Shell Shock

Pat Barker, *Regeneration* (1991)

On horror's head horrors accumulate.
—Shakespeare, *Othello*

Pat Barker's novel *Regeneration* fuses fact and fiction. It takes place in 1917, mainly at Craiglockhart hospital in Scotland, where the poet Siegfried Sassoon becomes the patient of the neurologist-psychiatrist Dr. W. H. R. Rivers. These two historical figures are surrounded by a group of fictional characters. What links them all is that they exhibit various forms of what was then known as shell shock.

"*Shell shock* is the war's emblematic psychiatric disorder,"[1] that is of World War I, the time of Barker's *Regeneration*. The term was applied to soldiers who suffered a breakdown as a consequence of their experiences under fire in modern warfare. Theories about its etiology shifted. At first it was taken literally as resulting from exposure to forces generated by high explosives with the vibrations or shock waves causing neurological disturbances. This view follows the precedent of hypotheses about what befell the victims of nineteenth-century railroad accidents.[2] Later this so-called "commotional shock" was thought to be accompanied by "emotional shock." Alternative descriptions of the same syndrome were "combat fatigue" and "war neurosis," the one more suggestive of a physical, the other more of a psychological condition. Shell shock was actually an amalgam of the physical and the psychological insofar as the fighting that the soldiers had undergone and the carnage they had witnessed led them to produce symptoms such as mutism, stammering, twitching, paralysis, nightmares, and hallucinations. So shell shock is a mode of speaking through the body, of converting fear and mental trauma into palpable manifestations.

Shell shock, Elaine Showalter argues in *The Female Malady*, was the male equivalent to the illness called hysteria in women. In a chapter titled

"Male Hysteria" (167–94), Showalter traces the great reluctance to acknowledge the possibility of the occurrence of hysteria in men, although Pierre Briquet (1796–1881) and subsequently both the great French neurologist Charcot and Freud had recognized it in males, admittedly far more rarely than in females.[3] The very phrase "shell shock," Showalter asserts, was a tolerated euphemism whose efficacy lay precisely in its capacity "to provide a masculine-sounding substitute for the effeminate associations of hysteria" (172).

Shell shock amounted to "a recategorization of behavior" from "cowardice" or "indiscipline" to "the belief that a particularly close hit by a heavy shell or a prolonged barrage prompted a mysterious transformation in the soldier's nervous system, which damaged his self-control."[4] While traditional-minded officers, who wished to enforce the military virtues of courage, honor, and duty, regarded the shell-shocked as "moral invalids," victims of war neurosis, as it also came to be known, were increasingly accorded the regard and sympathy that used to be reserved for the physically injured.[5] Still, in *Regeneration* patients allowed to go into town for a few hours' leave from the hospital are reluctant and ashamed to wear the yellow badge signifying their status. Their presumption that they are in disgrace contrasts with the automatic pity for the amputees that the character Madge glimpses on her visit to the hospital to see to her physically wounded fiancé.

Shell shock became an ever more serious problem as the war continued. Eric Leed cites an estimate in the *Official History of the War, Medical Services: Casualties and Medical Statistics*[6] that between 1916 and 1920 4 percent of the 1,043,653 British casualties were psychiatric cases.[7] The appearance of new cases after the end of hostilities is due to the amnesia and consequently delayed onset of the disorder now posited as one of its possible characteristic features.[8] After the war, around 65,000 British ex-soldiers were drawing disability because of "neurasthenia," 6 percent of the total, and 9,000 were hospitalized long-term.[9]

The nature of the combat in World War I was especially conducive to the development of shell shock. In the extended, inconclusive fighting in northern France and Flanders, the Allied and German armies went over the same ground again and again. Throughout October and November 1914 three battles raged in the mud at Ypres (Paschendaele) where the British casualties rose from 55,000 in the first encounter to 300,000 in the third. Even more protracted fighting took place on the Somme from July to November 1916, taking an equally heavy toll. By September 1916 tank warfare subsided into trench warfare, which put quite new strains on the troops. The siege-like situation in the trenches, in its combination of impersonality, randomness, and mechanized violence, was uniquely destructive to the combatants' psychic defenses by immobilizing them and making them feel disempowered as sitting targets. In chapter 5 of *No Man's land,* titled "Exit from the Labyrinth—Neurosis and War" (163–92), Eric Leed affirms the close association of "industrial warfare" and neurosis: "The dominance of long-range artillery, the machinegun, and barbed wire had immobilized combat, and immediately necessitated a passive stance of the soldier before the forces of mechanized slaughter. The cause of neurosis lay in the dominance of material over the possibilities of human movement" (164). This view is in keeping with the research carried out by the historical Dr. Rivers on the incidence of shell shock in the air force.[10] Rivers found war neurosis to be connected not to the intensity of the fighting nor to the length of service nor even to emotional predisposition, but to fixity, lack of active control. Pilots were less liable to war neurosis than were observers in the rear of the aircraft, and in the static balloon service psychic casualties outnumbered physical ones.

Medical opinion remained sharply divided throughout the war as to the most effective treatment, as Barker shows in *Regeneration.* The majority of physicians, suspecting the combatants of a self-protective malingering to save their lives, favored purely physical methods with the aim of quelling the symptoms and returning men to the front as quickly as possible. "Disciplinary" treatment, consisting of pain administration, usually by electrical apparatus, shouted commands, isolation, and limited rations, was based on conditioning principles and techniques derived from animal training. The patient's determination to hold on to his fixed ideas was pitted against the doctor's will to remove them by countersuggestion.

This mode of treatment is shown toward the end of *Regeneration* when the fictionalized Rivers pays a visit to London's leading neurological hospital in Queen Square. There he follows Dr. Lewis Yealland on his rounds and then witnesses the treatment of mutism by the application of a series of electrical shocks to the soldier's throat. The patient is not allowed to leave the room until he has uttered a few basic words. (The scene reproduces the historical Lewis Yealland's Case A 1, taken from his book, *Hysterical Disorders of Warfare,* excerpted in Allan Young's *Harmony of Illusions* [68]). Rivers is struck by the fact that in Yealland's ward "no questions were asked about their [the patients'] psychological state. Many of them, Rivers thought, showed signs of depression, but in every case the removal of the physical symptom was described as a cure" (*Regeneration,* 224). Nor does anybody know about either the suicide or the relapse rate. Yealland's brutal, mechanistic treatment attains, temporarily, the desired result of getting the men back to the front very rapidly. However, such methods were considered inappropriate for officers, whose problems were generally more complex, since they as commanders were supposed to be role models to their men.

Regeneration addresses this issue of the best way to handle shell-shocked officers. Dr. William Halse Rivers Rivers (1864–1922), who appears as the therapist in the novel, was not typical of the Royal Army Medical Corps because of his psychological orientation. A distinguished anthropologist as well as a psychiatrist, Rivers is now recognized as a pioneer in the psychological treatment of shell shock.[11] Rivers was exceptional in his time for his familiarity with Freud's work and his application of Freudian theory to the origins and treatment of the disorder. His 1917 article in *The Lancet* on "Freud's Theory of the Unconscious" affirms the supreme importance of *talking* over all aspects of the trauma underlying the symptoms rather than dealing solely with their surface manifestations as Yealland did.

Rivers's perception of war neurosis followed Freud in regarding the symptom as the key symbol of an internal drama that had its roots in especially horrifying events. In a seminal article in *The Lancet* of 2 February 1918, "The Repression of War Experience," Rivers advocates a radical departure from the then customary method of distraction as the optimal road to recovery. He cites the case of an officer disabled by insomnia and nightmares who "had been advised by everyone he had consulted, whether medical or lay, that he ought to banish all unpleasant and disturbing thoughts from his mind. He had been occupying himself for every hour of the day in order to follow this advice and had succeeded in restraining his memories and anxieties during the day, but as soon as he went to bed they would crowd upon him and race through his mind hour after hour, so that every night he dreaded to go to bed."[12] Rivers turned this approach upside down by encouraging the shell-shocked to *articulate* their haunting memories of the originating traumas so as to recuperate and ultimately exorcise them. Rivers also resorted to hypnosis, which enabled the patient to reenact the traumatic experience in the therapist's presence. Such reenactment could lead to the retrieval of the affect that had triggered the conversion. To bring back into the conscious mind the horrors that were being repressed and that needed to be confronted was a crucial step toward healing.

Rivers's choice of the term "repression" in the title of his article on war experience, together with his work on Freud's theory of the unconscious, clearly indicates that he was convinced of the centrality of the unconscious in the formation of war neuroses. However, despite several references to Freud and Freudian interpretations of dreams in *Regeneration,* Rivers was by no means a strict Freudian.[13] In his posthumously published volume, *Conflict and Dream* (1923), he defines those areas where he adheres to Freud and those where he diverges from him. He accepts Freud's fundamental conceptualization of dream work as consisting of condensation, displacement, plastic representation, and secondary elaboration, but is critical of the "tendency to lay undue stress on early factors and a relative neglect of recent conflicts, which I believe to be far more influential in the production of both dream and psycho-neurosis than is now usually supposed."[14] In according more weight to "the recency of the conflicts" than to the "wishes of early childhood" (104), Rivers puts into place the foundations for his understanding of war neuroses. The characteristic nightmares are a "direct negation of a wish" (68), a repetition without transformation of an experience that the dreamer had been trying in his waking state to keep out of his consciousness. Rivers envisaged the shell-shocked nightmare as "a faithful reproduction of some scene of warfare, usually some experience of a particularly horrible kind or some dangerous event . . . accompanied by an affect of a peculiarly intense kind" (66). Rivers grasped the emotional disturbance caused by warfare, and the need to resort to psychological treatments to alleviate the physically manifested distress. But partly because his psychological probing was a more protracted process than Yealland's coercion, it met with considerable skepticism from the authorities. In *Regeneration* one member of the Military Board screening men for their fitness to return to service reproaches Rivers: "What's he [the patient] want insight for? He's supposed to be killing the buggers, Rivers, not psychoanalyzing them" (245).

Rivers's *Conflict and Dream*, his article on "The Repression of War Experience," and Yealland's *Hysterical Disorders of Warfare* are among the works on which Barker draws for *Regeneration,* alongside Showalter's *Female Malady* and Leed's *No Man's Land.* Baker lists these sources in her brief "Author's Note" at the close of *Regeneration* (251–52) because "fact and fiction are so interwoven in this book" (251). Apart from Rivers and Yealland, a number of other characters cross over from history into the novel: the pacifist poet Siegfried Sassoon plays a major role, while his fellow poets Wilfred Owen and Robert Graves and the neurologist Dr. Henry Head, Rivers's prewar research partner in Cambridge, are subsidiary figures. The location of most of the action also bridges fact and fiction. Craiglockhart Military Hospital in the vicinity of Edinburgh, formerly a hydropathic establishment, was taken over by the Red Cross in 1916 as a hospital for shell-shocked officers. These historical strands are seamlessly interwoven with invented characters, mostly men traumatized by shell shock, although some of these too are based on cases chronicled by Rivers in "The Repression of War Experience" and *Conflict and Dream.* The foundations of *Regeneration* in such documentation enhance the credibility of the sometimes bizarre and often horrifying happenings recounted in the novel.

"Shell shock," together with "combat fatigue" and "war neurosis," has now been dropped from the vocabulary of psychiatry. In *DSM-I* (1952) the disorder appeared as "gross stress reaction," which was defined as a psychoneurotic disorder originating in an experience of intolerable stress. In *DSM-II* (1968) it is described as a "transient emotional disturbance." Only in *DSM-III* (1980) did shell shock acquire its current denomination as "post-traumatic stress disorder" (PTSD). The emergence of this separate diagnosis is traced by Young in *The Harmony of Illusions*, which is subtitled *The Invention of Post-Traumatic Stress Disorder*. In chapter 3, "The *DSM-III* Revolution" (89–117), Young argues that the "origins of the PTSD diagnosis are inextricably connected with the lives of American veterans of the Vietnam War, with their experiences as combatants, and later, as patients of the Veteran Administration (VA) Medical System" (108). The four diagnostic components of PTSD in *DSM-III* were a traumatic event, reexperiences of the event, numbing phenomena, and miscellaneous symptoms. Although PTSD is still associated primarily with the aftermath of warfare, in its recent reformulations it is applicable to responses to other stressful situations including prisoner-of-war or concentration camps, automobile and industrial accidents, the atomic bomb, rape, deadly floods or fires, and so on.

Like many other syndromes, PTSD underwent further elaboration and refinement in *DSM-IV* (1994). These are the current diagnostic criteria:

A. The person has been exposed to a traumatic event in which both of the following were present:
   (1) the person experienced, witnessed, or was confronted with an event or events that involved actual or threatened death or serious injury, or a threat to the physical integrity of self or others
   (2) the person's response involved intense fear, helplessness, or horror

B. The traumatic event is persistently reexperienced in one (or more) of the following ways:
   (1) recurrent and intrusive recollections of the event, including images, thoughts, or perceptions
   (2) recurrent distressing dreams of the event
   (3) acting or feeling as if the traumatic event were recurring (includes a sense of reliving the experience, illusions, hallucinations, and dissociative flashbacks, including those that occur on awakening or when intoxicated)
   (4) intense psychological distress at exposure to internal or external cues that symbolize or resemble an aspect of the traumatic event
   (5) physiological reactivity on exposure to internal or external cues that symbolize or resemble an aspect of the traumatic event

C. Persistent avoidance of stimuli associated with the trauma and numbing of general responsiveness (not present before the trauma), as indicated by three (or more) of the following:
  (1) efforts to avoid thoughts, feelings, or conversations associated with the trauma
  (2) efforts to avoid activities, places, or people that arouse recollections of the trauma
  (3) inability to recall an important aspect of the trauma
  (4) markedly diminished interest or participation in significant activities
  (5) feeling of detachment or estrangement from others
  (6) restricted range of affect (e.g., unable to have loving feelings)
  (7) sense of a foreshortened future (e.g., does not expect to have a career, marriage, children, or a normal life span)
D. Persistent symptoms of increased arousal (not present before the trauma), as indicated by two (or more) of the following:
  (1) difficulty falling or staying asleep
  (2) irritability or outbursts of anger
  (3) difficulty concentrating
  (4) hypervigilance
  (5) exaggerated startle response (427–28).

PTSD is a discrete entity in *DSM-IV*, not classified among the Somatization Disorders. This distinction is in conformity with *DSM-IV*'s overall tendency to increasing differentiation between syndromes in pursuit of greater scientific precision and in compliance with the demands of third-party insurers. Viewed from a broader perspective, however, PTSD clearly partakes of conversions from the mind into the body, denoted by "physiological reactivity." The mutism, profuse sweating, violent heart beating, and other exaggerated responses (for instance, to the sight of blood) are idioms of distress that devolve from and obliquely refer back to the originating traumatic event. Hindered by the sheer enormity of the repressed memory, those with PTSD avoid any type of recall and are therefore unable to air their suffering verbally. Instead they express it in a variety of phenomena that simultaneously mask and manifest the psychological undertow in physical form. In *The Harmony of Illusions* Young asserts that PTSD stems from the fusion of two types of pathogenic secrets: those of remembering (subconscious fixed ideas) and those of forgetting. "In one, the owner wants to hide the contents of his recollections from other people. In addition, he wants to forget the memory himself, or failing this, he wants to push it to the edges of awareness" (28). So it "remains unassimilated, a self-renewing presence reliving the moment of its origin" (29).

The entire range of PTSD symptoms is presented in *Regeneration* by the officers under Rivers's care at Craiglockhart. At dinner on the evening of his arrival Sassoon is struck by the fact that the meal takes place "in silence. The men on either side of him stammered so badly that conversation would have been impossible" (16). Stammering is widespread at Craiglockhart, and so are nightmares. As the men "shut the lid on memory" (33), by avoiding talk about their traumas during the day, at night they are haunted by those memories in their terrifying dreams, which they are also reluctant to divulge. Although the memories dog them relentlessly, they seek to evade them by silence, denial, repression, and distraction. They play golf and chess, watch funny films, scythe the high grass in the grounds, go for walks or occasionally into Edinburgh. In their conscious states, they make avoidance a way of life. Rivers's aim is to induce them to abandon that self-protective, but ultimately damaging, self-perpetuating stance by inducing them to recall and confront whatever had happened in hopes of defusing the associated anguish.

The wide spectrum of disturbances in PTSD is displayed in *Regeneration* through the variety of characters that appear in the novel. Some are minor, like Sassoon's roommate, Campbell, who suspects Sassoon of being a spy because of his first name. Rivers counters this rather ludicrous form of hypervigilance by tactfully giving it his consideration and then pointing out that German spies "*never* call themselves 'Siegfried'" (27). Another grotesque episodic figure is Featherstone, who flees the present by resorting to a stilted, mock-medieval kind of English. Broadbent is less devious, insistently requesting leave to visit his mortally sick mother—who subsequently turns up to see him. These peripheral cases provide a certain amount of comic relief to the grimmer experiences that predominate in *Regeneration*.

Apart from this incidental, background population of Craiglockhart, a few characters are developed in greater depth. While all of them exhibit features discussed by Rivers in "The Repression of War Experience," one of them, Burns, is taken directly from that article where he is described as "a young officer who was flung down by the explosion of a shell so that his face struck the distended abdomen of a German several days dead, the impact of his fall rupturing the swollen corpse. Before he lost consciousness the patient had clearly realised his situation and knew that the substance which filled his mouth and produced the most horrible sensations of taste and smell was derived from the decomposed entrails of an enemy. When he came to himself he vomited profusely and was much shaken, but carried on for several days, vomiting frequently and haunted by persistent images of taste and smell" (174). Burns is the most severely disabled at Craiglockhart. He is emaciated as a result of his constant vomiting, has noisy nightmares, and treks off alone into the wet countryside. Despite Rivers's gentle empathy, he fails to improve. Burns shows the inevitable limitations of Rivers' approach in certain cases. As Rivers concedes in his article: "It is not always, however, that the line of treatment adopted in these cases is so successful. Sometimes the experience which a patient is striving to forget is so utterly horrible or disgusting, so wholly free of any redeeming feature which can be used as a means of readjusting the attention, that it is difficult or impossible to find an aspect which will make its contemplation endurable" (174). Given an honorable discharge from the army, Burns retreats to his childhood home at the seaside, where Rivers goes to see him and saves him from a suicide attempt. The sense of a foreshortened future, of estrangement from others, of restricted affect, pronounced markers of PTSD, are translated by Burns into vomiting, insomnia, and nightmares.

The future is foreshortened too for Anderson, who worries about supporting his wife and son. A surgeon, Anderson admits that his "time in France has left [him] with a certain level of distaste for the practice of medicine" (29). This is a gross understatement. After carrying out countless amputations in the primitive conditions of a field hospital, Anderson has such a horror of blood that he falls totally apart at the sight of a few drops; when he cuts himself slightly while shaving, he weeps, screams, and wets himself. He tells Rivers of a nightmare in which he is thrown into a very dark carriage: "Like a grave. The first time I looked it was empty, but the next time you were there. You were wearing a post-mortem apron and gloves" (28). Rivers's incarnation here as a pathologist conveys Anderson's resentment at being dissected by the therapist. Even more significant is the earlier part of the same dream where Anderson sees himself facing his family naked, instead of in uniform, and running away from his father-in-law, who is chasing him through the bushes brandishing a big stick that has a hissing snake wound round it. The symbolism is transparent, with the snake signifying medicine, which Anderson is fleeing, stripped of his Royal Army Medical Corps uniform. The outcome for him is happier than for Burns: an administrative position in the medical section of the War Office that allows him to avoid blood permanently, yet still use his medical expertise, wear his uniform, and support his family.

The conversion into the physical domain is also quite evident in Willard, who has purple scars on his thighs and buttocks from injuries sustained when his company was retreating across a graveyard under heavy fire, and several tombstone fragments had become embedded in his flesh. The flesh wounds have healed, but Willard remains in bed or a wheelchair because he is convinced that he has an injury to the spine. Rivers finds no sign of any such injury, and tells Willard that he *can* walk. Willard angrily retorts that Rivers is accusing him of malingering or cowardice. Rivers gives a measured response: "'It's true paralysis occurs because a man wants to save his life. He doesn't want to go forward, and take part in some hopeless attack. *But neither is he prepared to run away.*' He smiled. 'Paralysis is no use to a coward, Mr. Willard. A coward needs his legs'" (112). Willard recovers, though not by means of insight; instead, he believes that Rivers has cured him physically of the spinal injury. This naive faith in Rivers is a way of saving face, but it also testifies to the healing power of the therapist's suggestions in what was clearly a psychosomatic disorder.

The therapeutic alliance comes to assume great force in the case of Billy Prior, the most extensively developed of the fictitious characters in *Regeneration*. From a working-class family, Prior has through determination, courage, and leadership qualities managed to become an officer. He has also concealed his debilitating asthma in order to be able to go to the front because he is ambitious and believes that those who have been in battle will stand the best chance of advancement in the postwar world. His initial stubborn mutism carries two possible implications. First it denotes his position midway between the classes since mutism was more frequent among common soldiers than in officers. More immediately, it signals his resistance to Rivers, whom he resents on social as well as professional grounds. Rivers had been a Cambridge researcher, a member of the educated, privileged class that Prior envies. And to be in need of psychiatric help strikes Prior not just as an indignity but as an insult to his self-image of independence and gallantry. By reading Rivers's book on anthropology and asking him questions, Prior both demonstrates his own intelligence and puts himself on a more equal footing with his therapist.

Even after he recovers the power of speech, Prior adamantly insists on his inability to remember anything. He does not believe that "talking *helps*. It just churns things up and makes them seem more real" (51). When Rivers argues that they are real and need to be faced, Prior replies: "[H]ow can I face them when I don't know what they are?" (51). Prior is obviously using forgetting for the purpose of avoidance. As Rivers tactfully explains to Prior's father (and to readers), "[P]erhaps there's something he's afraid to talk about, so he solves the problem by making it impossible for himself to speak. This is . . . beneath the surface. He doesn't *know* what he's doing" (56). Yet Prior had been a volunteer in the first week of the war. In this he fits the profile of the shell-shocked, as outlined by Grace Massonneu in her article "Social Analysis of a Group of Psychoneurotic Ex-Servicemen."[15] The overwhelming majority of them had been volunteers with a high sense of duty to the nation and idealistic expectations of war.

These expectations are one of the few subjects about which Prior does speak voluntarily, and on this matter he also dissociates himself from the officers. With overt contempt for "their *tiny tiny* minds," he tells Rivers of his realization that they had really believed "the whole thing's going to end in one big glorious *cavalry charge*" (66). This is confirmed by Niall Ferguson in his recent book, *The Pity of War*, where he characterizes the outlook in 1914 as "Britain's War of Illusions." The grandiose illusion[16] was shattered by the squalid realities of trench warfare. Rivers understands the impact of this imprisoning stasis, explaining to Prior that breakdown is not merely "a reaction to a single traumatic event. . . . It's more a matter of *erosion*. Weeks and months of stress in a situation where you can't get away from it" (105). Rivers's study of the men in observation balloons bears this out: "[I]t was prolonged strain, immobility and helplessness that did the damage" (222). The heroic adventure that enthusiastic volunteers had imagined turns out to be a sordid trial of endurance as they strive to survive, immobilized and disempowered, in the mud of the filthy trenches. In what were called "minor trench operations" 5,845 British soldiers were killed between December 1915 and June 1916.

Of the drama of such "minor" skirmishes Prior does have recall: "'I heard a shell coming. And the next thing I knew I was in the air, *fluttering* down . . .' He waved his fingers in a descending arc. 'I know it can't have *been* like that, but that's what I remember. When I came to, I was in a crater with about half a dozen of the men. I couldn't move my feet. I thought at first I was paralysed, but then I managed to move my feet. I told them to get the brandy out of my pocket, and we passed that round'" (79) But only under hypnosis is he able to reexperience the sensual impact of confinement in the tranches (101–4): "a dugout smell of wet sandbags and stale farts" (101), "the green, ratty, decomposing smell," "the chlorine-tasting tea," "crumbling parapets, flooded saps, dugouts with gagged mouths" (102). Two of his men, Sawdon and Towers, are "crouched over a small fire made out of shredded sandbags and candle ends" brewing tea and frying bacon for breakfast. Prior has not gone far before he hears a shell and a cry from another of his men, Landon: "Of the kettle, the frying-pan, the carefully tended fire, there was no sign, and not much of Sawdon and Towers either, or not much that was recognizable" (102). He and Landon shovel soil, flesh and splinters of blackened bone into a bag: "They'd almost finished when Prior shifted his position on the duckboards, glanced down, and found himself staring into an eye. Delicately, like somebody selecting a particularly choice morsel from a plate, he put his thumb and forefinger down through the duckboards. His fingers touched the smooth surface and slid before they managed to get a hold. He got it out, transferred it to the palm of his hand, and held it towards Logan. He could see his hand was shaking, but the shaking didn't seem to be anything to do with him. 'What am I supposed to do with this gob-stopper?'" (103). Feeling numbness all over his lower face, Prior is taken to a casualty clearing station, where he remembers that two of his men are dead. "Nothing else. Like the speechlessness, it seemed natural" (104).

In this climactic centerpiece to *Regeneration* Baker gives an unforgettably vivid evocation of both the gradually demoralizing and ultimately traumatic effect of trench warfare. The domestic details of the fire, the frying-pan, the tea, and the bacon are in sharp contrast to the sudden, violent destruction. Prior's shell shock is caused by the confluence of a lengthy period under chronic stress with the acute stress of picking up one of his men's eyes. The only way he can deal with these memories is by the avoidance of repression, and the only way to release him is through hypnosis by a therapist who has slowly won his trust and respect.

In contrast to Prior, Sassoon, whose arrival at Craiglockhart marks the beginning of *Regeneration*, is not actually suffering from shell shock. His hospitalization has been manipulated by his friend, Robert Graves, to keep scandal at bay after the publication of Sassoon's pacifist manifesto, "Finished with the War: *A Soldier's Declaration*," which forms a striking opening to the novel. While admitting that his statement is "an act of wilful defiance of military authority" (3), Sassoon pleads for the speedy end of warfare in favor of negotiation so as to spare the troops further suffering. Such a "*Declaration*" amounted to insubordination, exposing Sassoon to court martial and disgrace. To have him classified as shell-shocked and therefore not in full control of his thoughts and actions was a judicious escape from an embarrassing situation. The Military Board's sentencing of Sassoon to treatment at Craiglockhart thus represents another form of avoidance, this time on the part of the authorities. Shell shock was an expedient excuse.

So the concept of shell shock served a purpose in World War I that extended beyond individual into wider political needs. Neurotic symptoms were forefronted, as in Sassoon's case, as a compromise, for behind them "lay more dangerous possibilities, a more permanent neurosis, or a direct challenge to the war and those continuing it."[17] The breadth of the category of shell shock and its ambiguities afforded shelter for potential revolt and indiscipline as well as for genuine psychosomatic disorders. The passivity and impersonality intrinsic to trench warfare provided scant outlets for the aggressions and hostilities that built up among the troops. As the casualties rose to dizzying heights and the fighting covered the same ground over and again in futile, self-defeating destruction, the fear grew that improper targets such as the authorities or politicians would come under attack, as in Sassoon's "*Declaration*." Shell shock became a convenient explanation for any aberrant behavior, a more or less credible communal evasion of the real threat. The official report in the British Parliament on Sassoon's act deemed it a result of "nervous breakdown" (69).

Sassoon does have some symptoms of shell shock. He has had hallucinations of the sidewalk in Piccadilly strewn with corpses "clutching holes in their heads and waving their stumps around" (188). During his stay at Craiglockhart he awakes one day to a vision of Orme, his batman, come to rouse him for his watch. Only after a while does he remember that Orme is dead. Such an hallucinatory episode on awakening is characteristic of PTSD. Sassoon is also troubled by insomnia and nightmares. But, as Rivers notes at their first meeting over tea, he shows "no obvious signs of nervous disorder. No twitches, jerks, blinks, no repeated ducking to avoid a long-exploded shell" (10). However, Sassoon's deliberate courting of "*unnecessary* risks," which earned him the nickname "Mad Jack," is considered by Rivers as "one of the first signs of war neurosis" (12). And, as Graves points out to him later, he never talks about the future any more, making no plans, as if he expected to be killed. Rivers concludes that Sassoon has "a very powerful 'anti-war complex,'" which Graves interprets to mean that he is "*obsessed*" by the slaughter (198). Eventually Sassoon decides to return to the front, though without relinquishing his pacifist views. The figures in his nightmares make him feel guilty at being in the safety of Criaglockhart. Sassoon stands out in *Regeneration* as the nonavoider in both his "*Declaration*" and his resolve to return to battle in preference to accepting the comfortable training position he had been offered in England.

Regeneration is the story of Sassoon, beginning with his "*Declaration*" and closing on Rivers's notation "*Nov. 26, 1917. Discharged to Duty.*" Yet the interest in Rivers is at least as great, if not greater. As the therapist, he is the linchpin of the novel, linking the stories of the various patients at Craiglockhart. As the narrative progresses, the focus shifts increasingly onto Rivers's responses to the difficult dilemmas he repeatedly faces in regard not only to his patients but also to the clarification of his own attitude to the war. He becomes so exhausted by his workload at Craiglockhart that he is obliged to take a recuperative leave and then is persuaded by his old colleague, Dr. Henry Head, to accept the position of psychologist with the Royal Flying Corps at the Central Hospital, Hampstead, London, where he can deal with both physical trauma and war neurosis.

Is Rivers's leaving Craiglockhart an act of avoidance? That is unclear, for he will continue the same type of work in London, though perhaps he will not bear the responsibility of certifying men as fit to go back to the front. In some other respects, however, it is clear that he does resort to avoidance, like the officers under his care. He immediately recognizes in Sassoon's slightly slurred voice, with a flow of words sometimes hesitant, sometimes rushed, "a disguised stammer, . . . a life-long stammer" (10) because he himself struggles with the same speech impediment. Stammering, as Rivers explains to Prior, is parallel to mutism, which "seems to spring from a conflict between *wanting* to say something, and knowing that if you *do* say it the consequences will be disastrous" (96). Rivers adds that "it's usually thought that neurasthenic stammers arise from the same kind of conflict as mutism, a conflict between wanting to speak and knowing that w-what you've got to say is not acceptable" (97). With his customary impertinent familiarity, Prior replies: "Now that is lucky, isn't it? Lucky for you, I mean. Because if your stammer *was* the same as theirs—you might actually have to sit down and work out what it is you've spent fifty years trying not to say" (97).

One of the things that Rivers has been trying not to say throughout his life touches on his latent homosexuality. This is a secret he shares with Sassoon, who also has to conceal these tendencies because of the legal and social censure at the time. Graves tells Sassoon of a mutual friend who has been arrested for soliciting and of a rumor "of the existence of a German *Black Book* containing the names of 47,000 eminent people whose *private lives* make their loyalty to their country suspect" (204).18 The issue of homosexuality became particularly thorny during the war because of the danger of blackmail. On the other hand, as Graves comments, "in war you've got this *enormous* emphasis on love between men—comradeship— and everybody approves" (204). Prior, for instance, who appears to be bisexual, plays a quasi-maternal role toward his men at the front, as does Rivers toward his patients. In their domestic concern with their charges' physical welfare, both seem "more a sort of . . . *male mother*" (107). While Sassoon and Graves discuss the problem of homosexuality between themselves, Rivers does not speak of it other than obliquely, in his interest in a book that he and Sassoon had read about "the concept of an intermediate sex" (54).

Rivers is evasive about another deeply troubling question that Sassoon's presence raises in an acute form: the ethical conflict between his public and his private self. As an officer in the Royal Army Medical Corps, Rivers is under the obligation to cure his patients of shell shock, and if possible to send them back into active service, knowing full well that they may be maimed or killed. But even this public persona is bifurcated, since, as a physician, he is sworn to alleviate suffering and not to inflict further pain. Rivers winces literally and morally at the crude methods used by Yealland, who believes that patients have a more pressing obligation to the nation than to the survival of individuals. Rivers, on the other hand, with his acute sensitivity, is excruciatingly aware of the terrible costs of war, and tries in each case to weigh individual against social needs. Although he is relieved that Sassoon opts of his own accord to return to active duty, he is disturbed to find himself increasingly converted to Sassoon's pacifist convictions.

The phraseology in the novel is at this point much attenuated in comparison to Rivers's own words. Barker writes that "he was amused by the irony of the situation, that he, who was in the business of changing people, should himself have been changed and by somebody who was clearly unaware of having done it" (248–49). By contrast, Rivers's account of what he calls his "'Pacifist' Dream" in *Conflict and Dream* (165–80) reveals that the conflict that surfaced in this dream was far graver. He dreams of visiting a professor of physiology and a professor of another science, carrying two numbers of an Austrian anthropological journal in his Gladstone bag. The journal and the bag denote Rivers's dual interest in anthroplogy and medicine, the so-called Gladstone bag being traditionally carried by British doctors. That the journal is Austrian already hints at association with the enemy. This is reinforced by the fact that the professors are either Austrians or Germans; the sign on their door reads: "'Physiologisches Practicum'"[19] (Physiological Laboratory). To reach the laboratory door Rivers has turned to the right instead of to the left, as he had been instructed; he has departed from the prescribed route.

In the second part of the dream he is at lunch at the house of one of the professors, who has a German name. A fellow-guest is one of Rivers's patients, B, with whom he had previously talked about Germany. In Rivers's survey of the manifest content of the dream, he concludes that B stands for Sassoon: he "was not suffering from any form of psycho-neurosis, but was in the hospital on account of his adoption of a pacifist attitude while on leave from active service" (167). Rivers also recalls having just finished reading a book B had recommended, Barbusse's *Sous le feu* (*Under Fire*), a graphic, then famous evocation of warfare. He remembers clearly having "thought of the situation that would arise if my task of converting a patient from his 'pacifist errors' to the conventional attitude should have as its result my own conversion to his point of view. . . . Though my manifest attitude was definitely in favour of war to the finish, I had no doubt about the existence of a very keen desire that the war should end as soon as possible for the egoistic motive that I might get back to my proper studies" (168). In analyzing his dream, Rivers uncovers "a good opening for conflict and repression" (168). During the dream he thinks he is in uniform, but in the postdream analysis he is not sure of this, though sure that the German is in civilian dress. Rivers acknowledges that so long as he is in uniform, he is not a free agent in discussing pacifism with B. The severity of this conflict is attenuated in *Regeneration*. Perhaps the effect of this amendment is to make

Rivers seem more deeply in avoidance of his sympathy with Sassoon's pacifism.

Another dream is attributed to Rivers toward the end of the novel after his visit to Yealland's hospital. He sees himself in the electrical room, trying to apply an electrode to the patient, as Yealland had done. Unable to get it in, Rivers in his nightmare tries to force it: "[L]ooking down, he saw that the object he was holding was a horse's bit. He'd already done a lot of damage. The corners of the man's mouth were raw, flecked with blood and foam, but still he went on, trying to force the bit into the mouth, until a cry from the patient woke him" (236). On one level, this dream expresses Rivers's revulsion at Yealland's methods. Yet he perceives himself as doing the same thing. Putting a horse's bit into a man's mouth is an echo of Yealland's animalistic conditioning; horse-like foam as well as blood comes from the victim's mouth. But whereas Yealland's aim is to elicit speech, the effect of the horse's bit, an instrument of control, is to silence. Paradoxically, this nightmare suggests that at an unconscious level Rivers feels that he is squelching his patients' terrors even as he endeavors to get them to voice them.

Rivers' nightmare of the horse's bit leads into the very heart of *Regeneration*, the tension between silence and talking. In this respect PTSD resembles psychosomatic disorders in being a result of repression, not wanting to know, not articulating the causal distress. The themes of silence and talk are constantly reiterated motifs in *Regeneration*. It opens with a speech act, Sassoon's "*Declaration*," an enunciation of defiance. Having already made his beliefs public, Sassoon talks freely throughout, except for the barely perceptible stammer that indicates his real secret, his homosexuality.

Sassoon's fellow officers at Craiglockhart are in most cases reluctant to talk. Prior, with his mutism, is a prime example in his direct signal "NO MORE WORDS" (43); he can retrieve his crucial experience only under hypnosis because it is literally so unspeakably horrible. Burns is never able to speak of his trauma, and continues to convert into vomiting and avoidance of food. Uttering gibberish, as Fothergill does, is another way of sidestepping communication. Anderson, too, evades discussion of his revulsion from medicine by greatly understating its extent. Self-reproach plays some part in all the patients' repressive forgetting as a means of blocking out their sense of having failed as officers by breaking down. These men are as much unable to face themselves as their memories. Prior, whose origins are lower class, aptly describes the situation with a bluntness that the officers eschew: "They don't want the truth. It's like letters of condolence. 'Dear

Mrs. Bloggs, Your son had the side of his head blown off by a shell and took five hours to die. We did manage to give him a decent Christian burial. Unfortunately that particular stretch of ground came under heavy bombardment the day after, so George has been back to see us five or six times since then.' They don't want that. They want to be told that George—or Johnny—or whatever his name was—died a quick death and was given a decent send off" (134).

In the context of this pervasive avoidance, it seems paradoxical that *Regeneration* abounds in dialogue. There is discussion between Rivers and his superior at Craiglockhart, Bryce, about the patients' condition and the running of the institution. Mostly there is dialogue between Rivers and each of his patients individually. These exchanges are, however, often punctuated by silences on both sides. The men either maintain that they don't remember beyond a certain point, or even say, like Prior, "I don't want to talk about this" (96). Interestingly, Rivers, too, is notorious for his long silences. They occur not in ordinary conversation, as with Bryce or the members of the Craiglockhart staff or even of the Military Board, but in the therapeutic sessions. Contrary to his horse'a bit dream of coercion, he refrains from pressing or bullying his patients, as Yealland does. His silences testify to his restraint, patience, and empathy. When he visits Burns at his seaside home, he deliberately doesn't mention Burns's evident idiosyncracies, partly because Burns is no longer technically his patient, but primarily because he respects him enough to wait for him to initiate the matter if he so wishes. With the men who are his patients at Craiglockhart, Rivers has the professional responsibility of trying to help them to break out of their silence and repression. His own silences project tact as well as his understanding of their reticence because like them he avoids things he doesn't want to face, let alone say.

Does speaking out about painful memories then effect regeneration? The model is derived from the experiment Rivers had conducted before the war in Cambridge, severing and suturing his colleague, Dr. Henry Head's radial nerve and charting the progress of its regeneration over a period of five years. The process is painful, and we are not told whether the nerve ever heals completely. In a transferral from the physical to the psychological that is a reversal of the process of somatization, regeneration is posited as the product of developing the capacity to confront and articulate the trauma. Rivers attributes Sassoon's "early and rapid recovery" to his "determination to remember" (26). On the whole, those who do manage to talk, like Prior, regenerate, whereas those like Burns and Anderson, who cannot speak, remain captive to their symptoms.

Where Rivers himself stands along this spectrum of avoidance/openness is one of the most fascinating aspects of *Regeneration*. In the course of the novel, he sickens under the overload of his responsibilities and the stressful nature of his work. It is as if he in turn sustained a war neurosis, especially as he comes secretly to share Sassoon's pacifist convictions. He recalls that *"Physician, heal thyself"* (106) had been one of his father's favorite texts. In a night of rain and wind, when he knows that his patients are thinking of their battalions sinking ever deeper into the mud, he gets "all the familiar symptoms. Sweating, a constant need to urinate, breathlessness, the sense of blood not flowing but squeezing through his veins. The slightest movement caused his heart to pound" (139). To Bryce he briskly diagnoses his attack as "psychosomatic" (140). Even after he leaves Criaglockhart to visit his brother, he awakes "suffering from the usual medley of physical and neurasthenic symptoms—headaches, dry mouth, pounding heart" (156).

Later, Head reproaches Rivers for all his *"self-laceration"* (240), a trait that emerges most clearly from his dream about the horse's bit. He recognizes its dominant affect as "self-reproach," the awareness of being *"locked in"* every bit as much as his patients, of being "in the business of controlling people," and of silencing his patients by getting them to overcome the protest of their unconscious represented in their conversion symptoms. He believes that the demands made on him at Craiglockhart had changed him from "being reticent, introverted, reclusive," and that particularly his encounter with Sassoon's rebellion had forced him "into conflict with the authorities over a very wide range of issues . . . medical, military. Whatever" (249). The suspension points and "Whatever" surely suggest "sexual." And so Rivers is shown to persist in his own (probably at least partly necessary at the time) repression and avoidance.

Regeneration differs from the majority of literary portrayals of psychosomatic disorders in devoting as much attention to the healer as to the patients. The closest parallel is with *The Strange Case of Mademoiselle P.,* where Dr. Mesmer's thoughts preponderate in quantity and intensity over those of his young patient. In both instances this distribution of readers' interest is determined by the disposition of the narrative: the focalization is more through the physician than the patient(s). In O'Doherty's novel this is readily apparent, since three of the five sections are first-person accounts by Mesmer. In *Regeneration* the viewpoint shifts with greater flexibility, but the dominating intelligence is that of Rivers. His dilemmas and his tendency to psychosomatic conversion make him a riveting figure. His own problems heighten his sensitivity as a healer through his instinctive empathy with his patients, yet in the long run such empathy undermines the detachment he needs, and so leads to burn-out.

The sharing of the spotlight between patients and therapist is not the only respect in which *Regeneration* departs from the pattern common to images of psychosomatic disorders in literary texts. Generally, as in *Broken Glass* and *The Strange Case of Mademoiselle P.,* it is one character who displays symptoms, although in *Buddenbrooks* the proclivity to conversion extends beyond the family member branded "the sore spot" to his siblings. In *Regeneration,* by contrast, the patients form a cluster, a group at once unified and particularized. As veterans and victims of combat, all the men at Craiglockhart are alike. The etiology of their disorders is the same, a repression of the traumas they have undergone; all readily fit the diagnosis of PTSD, and all exhibit its salient symptomatology. However, within this fundamental community, Barker succeeds in drawing sharply distinctive profiles of the men institutionalized together. Sassoon's pacifism, Burns's intractable vomiting, Anderson's panic at the sight of blood, Prior's mutism, Campbell's hypervigilance, Fothergill's quaint locutions distinguish the members of the group. Through this vivid individualization Barker achieves a group portrait of PTSD in *Regeneration* that is at once singular as well as typical in its overall outlines.

In the context of the disorders, too, *Regeneration* differs from most of the other works, where the setting and the conflict are most commonly familial. Here the social environment is communal: the trenches or the hospital. These milieux are shown to spawn a certain amount of interpersonal dissonance through the closeness forced onto the men. In the trenches conflicts are held in check by the rigid hierarchy of military authority as well as the shared danger; in the hospital, on the other hand, they are expressed in repeated complaints about roommates' disruptive behavior. Sporadic outbursts of anger, characteristic of PTSD, are signs of the tensions among the patients at Craiglockhart.

But these interpersonal frictions, which are so central to *Broken Glass, The Strange Case of Mademoiselle P.,* and *Buddenbrooks,* are marginal in *Regeneration,* in which the core problems are essentially intrapersonal. None of these men, except Sassoon, can on their own resolve their conflicted feelings about their war experiences. They have been exposed to events far over and above the normal limits of human endurance, yet as officers they have expected of themselves a superhuman endurance. Their disappointment at their failure is to some small extent blunted by their conversions into their bodies. A physical injury is more acceptable than a psychological breakdown, which is perceived as weakness, or at the very least a shortfall from the ideals and self-image these officers have been conditioned to cherish.

The psychological substratum to the psychosomatic disorders in this novel is never in any doubt. Shell shock is directly triggered by the ghastliness of what these men have witnessed. *Regeneration* therefore departs again from the format common to many literary portrayals of psychosomatic disorders, that of the mystery to be probed. The emphasis in *Regeneration* is less on the detection of broad causalities, although Rivers aims in his therapeutic interactions with his patients to draw them to the point where they can retrieve onto the conscious level the specific experiences they want to push aside. The assumption motivating the treatment of psychosomatic disorders is the same in *Regeneration* as in the other works, namely, that conscious recognition and understanding of the formative factors underlying the conversion will result in its dissipation. Yet, as Rivers grants in his article "Repression in War Neurosis," the method is not invariably successful. It is successful with Prior but not with Burns. *Regeneration* is more skeptical in its suppositions about cure than many other works, where recovery follows on conscious cognition, whereas continuing denial perpetuates the condition.

This refusal to simplify is one reason for *Regeneration*'s resistance to neat closure. It is enfolded in the story of Sassoon, opening on Rivers's and Bryce's reading of Sassoon's "*Declaration*" and ending with Rivers's notation of his discharge from Craiglockhart. But Sassoon's fate still remains undetermined, for there is a fair likelihood that he will perish in the warfare. Only from the vantage of hindsight—and the "Author's Note" (251)—do we learn that he survived, dying a natural death in 1967. Wilfred Owen, however, fell in 1918. The stories of Prior and Rivers are left still more open, to be continued in the second and third volumes of the trilogy. Prior is the pivotal figure in *The Eye in the Door* and appears again in *The Ghost Road*, toward whose dramatic finale he is killed in battle. Rivers, too, is prominent in both subsequent novels, especially in *The Ghost Road*, where the high fever of an attack of Spanish 'flu instigates his hallucinatory memories of his adventures as an anthropologist among head hunters, experiences that form a parallel to those of war. In *The Ghost Road*, too, Sassoon's pacifism is reinforced in Rivers' mind by the devastating final verdict of Hallett, a very young officer, who has been grotesquely wounded and who lingers in an agonizing death. Rivers is the only one able to understand what Hallett tries to say through that part of his mouth that has not been blasted away: "'It's not worth it.'"[20] So the trilogy is ultimately rounded out by a painful validation of the pacifist position on which it had begun.

The trilogy represents a meditation on war and its inevitable costs. Among those costs are psychosomatic disorders, as damaging though perhaps less immediately striking than physical injuries. The illnesses of the men at Craiglockhart are situated in the large context of the ever present frame of the war. These patients have been swept up into international political hostilities over which the individual has no control. Sassoon's stand, however courageous, is rendered pretty futile by the authorities' manipulations to minimize its impact by labeling him as shell-shocked. While Sassoon is able to fashion a compromise by returning to the front and still uphold his pacifist principles, his fellow officers are trapped in intrapersonal conflicts stemming not from innate personal psychological problems but precipitated by immediate external factors such as the stresses of trench warfare. Their traumas and their symptoms are, as Rivers insists, "REAL" (140), but they are in some cases, such as those of Burns and Anderson, beyond remediation because of the intensity of the horror that provoked them.

Regeneration therefore not only resists closure but also questions the common belief that psychosomatic disorders are amenable to resolution or amelioration by uncovering their unconscious sources through psyche-searching talk. The novel is so challenging and rewarding precisely because of its ingrained ambivalences. Sassoon, the pacifist, goes back to the front; Rivers, the therapist whose duty it is to fit men for resuming combat, is increasingly dubious of the legitimacy of his work as he comes to be converted to Sassoon's views; what is more, the proponent of innovative treatment of shell shock by confrontation and verbalization of the horror has to acknowledge that his approach does not always work. And he fears, as his horse's bit dream reveals, that "*he* silenced *his* patients" (238). Is this just an erosion of his self, occasioned by stress and exhaustion, similar to that suffered by his patients? or do his efforts to prompt talk paradoxically lead to a further masking of his patients' "unwitting protest" (238), a mere displacement of affect into language rather than a genuine release from horror? It is interesting that the novel begins with a speech act and ends with a silent entry into Sassoon's file.

Regeneration is the most complex literary portrayal of psychosomatic disorders of the texts I discuss in this book. Apart from grafting fiction onto fact, it also blends the real with the almost surrealistic in the incidents from warfare such as Prior's touching the eye and Burns's ingestion of decomposed flesh. Foremost among its subtle fusions is the tension between, on the one hand, Rivers's penetrating understanding of the mechanisms of psychosomatic disorders and his professional billiance, and, on the other hand, his half-repressed self-doubting. Barker has produced a hauntingly impressive, forceful picture of PTSD as a conjunction of unconscious avoidance, guilt, and self-censure.

CHAPTER ELEVEN

Outing the Distress

Hasn't she gone off her head? I don't mean metaphorically, I mean in the strict medical sense
——Dostoevsky, *The Idiot*

The essence of psychosomatic disorders lies in the outing of an unacknowledged psychological distress through the body. What forms does
this outing take in the body of literature about such disorders? Specifically,
how do the medical and the imaginative writing relate to each other? In
what ways does the "metaphoricity" of the literary works modify and aug-
ment "the strict medical sense"?[1] I would like to argue that the two types of
writing complement and supplement each other. The long-standing Psychiatry and Literature reading group at the University of North Carolina at
Chapel Hill, for example, is based on the belief that the discussion of literary works is useful to psychiatrists.

In drawing comparisons between the two modes of writing about psychosomatic disorders, one fundamental caveat has to be made. Both medical and imaginative writing on this topic are subject to wide variations.
Medical thinking has shifted radically in the past 150 years in a complex,
nonlinear course. The range of the creative literature is equally great. Yet
each type of writing forms an entity with quite distinctive characteristics
that legitimate a broadly based comparison.

The medical writings are governed by a necessarily practical purpose:
that of identifying the signs of diverse syndromes as a preliminary to initiating the appropriate remediation. The implicit belief systems over the past
century and a half or so span far-reaching transformations: from humoral
medicine through Mesmeric and Freudian approaches to behavioristic,
psychopharmacological, and neuroimmunological methods. However, the
overarching thrust remains constant: to establish, according to the ideas of
each time, the universally valid paradigms thought to underlie the overt
symptoms. Within the parameters of each school—humoral, Mesmerian,

Freudian, behavioristic, psychopharmacological, neuroimmunological—
the fundamental aim is the same: to grasp the particular nature of patients'
problems, to define and demarcate them in order to choose the optimal
means to cure or palliate them.

In this succession of epistemologies, the imaginative literature meshes
directly with the beliefs dominant at each period. Roger Chillingworth in
The Scarlet Letter, whose action takes place in the mid-seventeeth century,
subscribes to the tenets of humoral medicine in his acceptance of the
"strange sympathy betwixt soul and body." In the mid-nineteenth century,
when somatic medicine was decisively in the ascendant, Dr. Grabow, the
experienced physician in *Buddenbrooks,* is shown to be totally at a loss how
to deal with Christian's bewildering series of complaints. *The Strange Case of
Mademoiselle P.,* set in 1777, endorses on the surface Mesmer's magnetism,
letting it overlap with the unmistakable Freudian undercurrent. Freud's
insights buttress the approach to post-traumatic stress disorder during
World War I in *Regeneration* by Dr. Rivers, who was, like Freud himself, both
a neurologist and a psychiatrist. By the late 1930s, in *Broken Glass,* the role
of intuitively wise counselor has been assumed by the shrewd family doctor.
So each of these literary works depicts the normative mode of handling a
psychosomatic disorder at the historical moment of its action. Granted that
Mesmer is conflated with Freud in *The Strange Case of Mademoiselle P.,* and
that Dr. Rivers in *Regeneration* is a pioneer, the congruence between the
medical epistemology of each period and the practices incorporated into
the literary portrayals is still quite extensive and persuasive.

But the literary works diverge from the development of medical writing in their continuing portrayal of essentially humanistic approaches, as
exemplified by Dr. Hyman in *Broken Glass* and Dr. Rivers in *Regeneration.*
Their empathetic stance toward their patients and their colorful repartee
contrasts with the markedly flat and repetitive language of *DSM-IV.* Its purpose is to assure maximum standardization so as to facilitate that collation
of symptom clusters crucial to differential diagnosis. The diagnostician projected by *DSM-IV* seeks to maintain as detached and dispassionate a gaze as
possible in the task of assessing the patient, although some degree of subjective impression is inevitable in psychiatric evaluation. However, *DSM-IV*
seems to imply that such input is undesirable by advocating strict adherence to severely delimited lists of criteria. The emphasis is more on
patients' behavior than on their emotions. Their relationship to their environment, a factor so central to Engel's biopsychosocial model, is relatively
little heeded. The cost of the scientific precision of *DSM-IV* is a reification
of the patient into an amalgam of symptoms that amount to a syndrome;
the human being is effaced in favor of the disorder.

The method of *DSM-IV* is justifiable only by its status as a heuristic diagnostic tool, but it has spawned a proclivity to depersonalization that

extends beyond the diagnostic phase. The ideal of exactitude in the name of scientific rigor is equally apparent in most of the articles in the journal *Psychosomatic Medicine*. While the researchers do pay more attention to their subjects' social settings, for example by examining the impact of significant others' attitudes in certain disorders, they present their findings in elaborate statistical tables that document the averages and the medians, thereby turning the individual into an abstraction. The loss is especially disturbing in relation to psychosomatic disorders, where so much hinges on what Lipowski calls "perception and cognition," that is, the individual's reaction to circumstances. What is deeply distressing to one person may hardly touch another.

Not all current psychiatric writing is of such austerity. *Psychosomatic Medicine* itself publishes articles that argue for the more humanistic view that patients are not merely "collections of organs, cells, molecules, ions, and so forth but also individuals."[2] One recent contributor opposes the relegation of psychological factors in *DSM-III* and *IV* as "merely ancillary elements" and points to "the remarkable difficulty of many psychosomatic patients in finding words to describe feelings."[3] This is an important observation, for it is frequently patients' incapacity to verbalize distressing feelings that is the root of conversion disorders. But this characteristic on the part of patients is completely overlooked in *DSM-IV*. By contrast, the *Synopsis of Psychiatry* (ed. Kaplan, Sadock, and Grebb) occasionally includes cameo case histories that illustrate not just the symptoms themselves but the situations in which they have typically occurred.

The sparseness and abstraction of late twentieth-century conventions of psychiatric discourse are thrown into relief by juxtaposition with the evocative richness of Freud's case histories. Freud embeds his patients in their family and social context, conceiving their intrapsychic conflicts as intimately connected to their interpersonal dilemmas. He reconstructs imaginatively—sometimes arguably *too* imaginatively, as in the case of Dora—the elements involved in the origins of their complaints. In thus switching from traditional neurology to innovative, indeed revolutionary psychoanalysis, Freud himself was troubled by the likelihood, at an early and precarious stage in his career, "dass die Krankengeschichten, die ich schreibe, wie Novellen zu lesen sind" ("that the case histories I write read like stories"); he feared "dass sie sozusagen des ernsten Gepräges der Wissenschaftlichkeit entbehren" ("that they lack, so to speak, the serious imprint of scholarship").[4] Freud here delineates a tension, even an antagonism between serious scientific scholarliness and narratology.

Narratology is held up by the neurologist-writer Oliver Sacks as the counterbalance to the "defectology" that is the usual practice in medicine in its endeavor to diagnose and wherever possible to remedy the patient's defects.[5] Sacks outlines the routine sequence of objective testing and clinical observation in relation to each of the neurological cases he describes in *The Man Who Mistook His Wife for a Hat* and *An Anthropologist on Mars*. Yet he comes to realize that the testing alone captures merely one aspect of his idiosyncratic patients, namely their departure from the norm. Only a totally different perception can do justice to them as human beings.

The best example of this dichotomy is the "painfully shy and with-drawn" Rebecca, who "had a partial cleft palate, which caused a whistling in her speech; short, stumpy fingers, with blunt, deformed nails; and a high, degenerative myopia requiring very thick spectacles."[6] Sacks sets his negative, medical first impression of her against his second, quite different view. When he first sees her in the clinic and applies the standard tests to her, he registers her "merely or wholly, as a casualty, a broken creature, whose neurological impairments I could pick out and dissect with precision" (180). The next time he sees her, it is outside the clinic on a lovely spring day, and Rebecca is "sitting on a bench, gazing at the April foliage quietly, with obvious delight. Her posture had none of the clumsiness which had so impressed me before. Sitting there, in a light dress, her face calm and slightly smiling, she suddenly brought to mind one of Chekov's young women—Irene, Anya, Sonya, Nina—seen against the backdrop of a Chekovian cherry orchard. . . . This was my human, as opposed to my neu-rological vision" (180). Remembering her "warmly" (177), Sacks pleads for the importance of narratology as a corrective to defectology.

A parallel instance is Martin, a sixty-one-year-old man with brain damage and intellectual limitations but such an extraordinary musical retentiveness that Sacks calls him "A Walking Grove" after Grove's immense, nine-volume *Dictionary of Music and Musicians*, which Martin knows by heart. Like Rebecca, he is at one level a disaster, "often childish, sometimes spiteful, and prone to sudden tantrums. . . . He sniffed, he was dirty, he blew snot on his sleeve—he had the look (and doubtless the feel-ings) at such times of a small, snotty child" (190). However, he becomes "a different man" once "he returned to song and church" (191). In pinpoint-ing Rebecca's and Martin's deficits, Sacks resorts to such technical terms as "apraxias," "agnosias," "cerebral achromatopsia," and "cystoid macular edema" to give a precise medical designation to their impairments. But he partners this defectology with a rare capacity for narratology that restores to Rebecca and Martin their human essence, their "poignant innocence, transparency, completeness, and dignity" (174).

The situation of those exhibiting conversion disorders is in certain respects quite different from that of Rebecca and Martin who suffer from clearly established neuropathologies. The variegated symptoms of psycho-somatic disorders, on the other hand, largely resist recognizable patterns. There is no medically ascertainable reason for the sudden paralysis of

Sylvia's legs in *Broken Glass,* or for Marie-Therese's blindness in *The Strange Case of Mademoiselle P.,* or for Christian's inability in *Buddenbrooks* to swallow a peach. Nor do the combat veterans in *Regeneration* have actual damage to their bodies, although some of them believe so in an attempt to save face. The type of defectology applicable to Rebecca and Martin proves unfruitful in conversion disorders because the body is not the true site of the problem, only a displacement substitute. For this reason the defectology exemplified in *DSM-IV* does not capture the essence of psychosomatic disorders, recording only their surface manifestations. In "the strict medical sense" nothing ails those with conversion disorders, as Barbour discovered when patients came to Stanford's Diagnostic Clinic with sheaves of X rays and test results that had yielded no answers to their complaints. His experience is evidence of the failure of defectology in psychosomatic disorders.

Under these circumstances, narratology becomes a necessity as the sole effective path to both medical understanding and the patient's self-understanding. As the principle animating the free associative talk of psychoanalysis as well as of its successor, psychotherapy, narratology enables the individual to engage in self-exploration and self-clarification under the astute guidance of a trained listener. Narratology is deeply implicated too in the metaphoricity at work when the inner distress is outed as a bodily complaint, for in effect the patient is indirectly divulging her or his suffering. Only by reversing that conversion, by recuperating the originating subconscious distress into a conscious, cohesive narrative can the disorder be dispelled. The classic example of such a resolution is the case of Freud's patient, Cäcilie, who for years had attacks of intractable facial pain that were not alleviated by any medical means, yet that dissipated when she recalled—and spoke of—the slap in the face which was turned into the metaphoric neuralgia. The adjective "metaphoric" does not imply that Cäcilie did not feel *real* pain, although it was caused not by a bad tooth or a sinus infectiom, but a sense of psychological hurt made manifest symbolically.

In the case of Cäcilie, as of the literary patients I have discussed, it is the *absence* of narratology that induces the conversion disorder. All the characters have, deliberately or unwittingly, guarded a silence intended to be self-protective but that proves in fact to be self-damaging. Therein lies the major irony intrinsic to psychosomatic disorders: that the very maneuver meant to be protective inverts into the injurious. This protection is supposed to be vouchsafed through the silence all the characters maintain about the various secrets they harbor: marital/sexual secrets in *Broken Glass,* family secrets in *Buddenbrooks* and *The Strange Case of Mademoiselle P.,* guilt secrets in *The Scarlet Letter, Thérèse Raquin,* and *Regeneration.* While these categories may overlap, the secrets withheld from the conscious mind always function as a form of self-censorship, a defense mechanism that mis-fires. For, as Freud pointed out, it is the *miscarriage* of repression that underlies the conversion.[7] When the distress cannot be totally banished, it is supplanted, that is, converted into the body. The unsuccessful effort to avoid a distress that is feared and intuited though unavowed becomes a dis-guised idiom of distress. So it serves at once as a manifestation *and* a mask, a substance *and* a shadow, a fact *and* a fiction. The metaphor bridges biol-ogy and psychology.

Just as silence and the associated repression trigger conversion disor-ders, their opposite, narration, can be the agency of release and healing. Many of the literary works reveal the link between genuine self-scrutiny, the candid confrontation of the problem previously avoided, and healing release from the symptom. Once the secret is retrieved into the conscious mind, brought into the open in the form of words, its potential for psy-chological harm is attenuated or even abolished. This is most evident in *Broken Glass* as Sylvia, under Dr. Hyman's persistent prompting and ques-tioning, finds her own voice and the confidence to give utterance to what has been troubling her; when she can speak out about what she could not stand psychologically, she is able again to stand on her legs. The play hinges on the metaphoricity of physical standing as the cipher for standing in the sense of being able mentally to bear.

In other instances, the outcome is less clear-cut, although the pattern of struggle between silent repression and voiced narration recurs. *The Strange Case of Mademoiselle P.* shows the coincidence of recovery and speech as Marie-Therese regains vision under Mesmer's treatment at the same time that she assumes voice in the novel's central section. But after she is made to return to her parents' house and duress, she relapses into blind-ness and into silence too. Among the men at Craiglockhart in *Regeneration*, Sassoon is conspicuous for actually publishing his *Declaration;* his convic-tion of the necessity for speaking out overrides the threat such an action poses to his reputation and position. Although he has been exposed to the horrors of warfare, he does not develop full-blown PTSD because, instead of avoiding the memories, he outs them in a verbal protest. In contrast to Sassoon, Prior is at first mute and for long sparing with words; he is enabled to recount his traumatizing experience only under hypnosis, a subterfuge that allows him to speak out in a kind of trance, which both mitigates his responsibility for his words and blunts his mixture of revulsion, survivor guilt, and shame at what he has to tell. Despite his resistances, his resent-ments, and his rancor, Prior does emerge from PTSD to go back to the front eventually. Not so Burns, whose defining trauma was literally so unut-terably gross that he cannot bear to revisit it by verbalization; he remains locked into unspeakable memories.

The other figures whose conversion disorders are irreversible and who end badly share with Burns an absence of narratology. Dimmesdale in *The Scarlet Letter* is constrained by both powerful external, societal pressures and internal inhibitions from publicly talking about his guilt. Until his last moments Dimmesdale feels obligated to uphold his façade and therefore to maintain silence. By contrast, Christian Buddenbrook, with his endless lamentations, is to all appearances an overtalker, but he lives in a society that prizes tight-lipped stoicism, refuses to heed his diatribes, condemning them with as much self-righteous contempt as is provoked by his noncon- formist behavior. So for all his torrents of words, Christian is shut into his distress with nothing but recriminatory listeners who reinforce his solipsis- tic isolation. As for Thérèse and Laurent in *Thérèse Raquin,* they are por- trayed as essentially inarticulate, unable to express feelings other than through body language. The shortfall in narratology in these cases is a deci- sive impediment to the possibility of healing.

If narratology well serves the protagonists, so too it does readers. For it is eminently conducive to the elaboration of the biopsychosocial model that gives a broad perspective on the origins and unfolding of the disorder up to the critical point of its full crystallization into a defect. All the literary works contextualize the sufferers in relation to their environment, pre- senting its physical features as a metaphor for its moral atmosphere. The stern New England Puritan religiousness in *The Scarlet Letter,* the grim dep- rivation in *Thérèse Raquin,* the austere North German Protestant work ethic in *Buddenbrooks,* the anti-Semitism in *Broken Glass,* the court's hypocrisy in *The Strange Case of Mademoiselle P.,* the horrors of trench warfare in *Regener- ation:* knowledge of all these factors, so graphically evoked, contributes to readers' understanding of the processes of unconscious rebellion as well as of defense in the characters' interactions with family and milieu in ways that promote conversion disorders. Silhouetted against their background, the sufferers assume a vivid, multidimensional wholeness that is beyond the purview of medical texts. Literary works thus compensate for what has been lost through the disappearance of the individual, humanistic case history exemplified by Freud's "stories."

In addition to social spaciousness, literary works also have the advan- tage of a temporal expansiveness that permits the tracing of the growing interpersonal frictions and intrapsychic conflicts. There are two main modes of handling time: the long, chronologically articulated duration, or the opening up from the start in the present crisis onto a retrospective assessment of the past. Temporal along with social capaciousness is most to the fore in *Buddenbrooks,* where the action extends from 1835 to 1875, and is punctuated by frequent references to specific dates that act as markers of the passage of the years. *The Scarlet Letter,* though less directly concerned with time than *Buddenbrooks,* also encompasses a considerable number of years. A variant on such protracted chronology occurs in *The Strange Case of Mademoiselle P.*, in which the first four sections take place within a brief span in 1777, while the last one, dating from 1814, records Mesmer's recollections of what had happened earlier. Thus the novel combines the two modes of organizing time in its simultaneous forward and backward movement. *Thérèse Raquin*, too, is primarily linear in its progression from adultery through murder to suicide over a relatively short segment of about a couple of years, although it also looks backward in the life histories of Thérèse and Laurent. The retrospective that provides a partial motivation for the action in *Thérèse Raquin* is crucial to the other two works, *Broken Glass* and *Regeneration*, in which the protagonists' current state of crisis is gradually exposed through exploration of their past experiences. But whether the time line is progressive or retrospective, the ultimate effect is the same. For the opportunity given to readers to observe the changes wrought in the characters by their actions and their reactions to circumstances and events affords insight into the causes and onset of the disorders to which they fall prey. Factors that might emerge in the course of psychotherapy are clearly outed in the literary works in a manner that fosters understanding of the processes of somatization.

The possibilities for understanding are likewise heightened by the literary works' aptitude for showing characters' thoughts, either in the first person or through dialogic utterances. Admittedly, such a procedure can be a two-edged sword, on account of the bias innate to the subjective view. However, at issue here are not the facts as objective truths but the individual's "cognition and perception" of the situation, an important variable in the evolution of psychosomatic disorders. Whether the sufferer's vision is correct or skewed is immaterial; it is the cogency of that vision for that person that is decisive, and this is an aspect that a literary work can forcefully convey. For example, Christian Buddenbrook is most unlikely to die by swallowing a peach stone. We as readers realize this, but by witnessing his panic, we also realize the validity of belief in that scenario. Despite our perhaps ironical or even cynical detachment, we are enabled better to grasp the state of mind of those in the grip of such a conversion disorder. Through its use of metaphor the literary work outs the distress inherent in the situation. What Christian cannot "swallow" is the life expected of him any more than Sylvia in *Broken Glass* can "stand" hers.

The metaphoricity of illness has been described by Susan Sontag in the phrase: "One's mind betrays one's body."[8] She cites Kafka's comment in his letter to his friend, Max Brod, in 1917 when he was diagnosed with the tuberculosis that was to kill him: "Manchmal scheint es mir, Gehirn und Lunge hätten sich ohne mein Wissen verständigt. 'So geht es nicht weiter' hat das Gehirn gesagt und nach fünf Jahren hat sich die Lunge bereit erklärt, zu helfen" (Sometimes it seems to me as if my mind and my lungs had communicated without my knowledge. "Things can't go on like this," my mind said, and five years later my lungs declared themselves ready to help out).[9] Kafka here conceives his illness as a way out of his distress, casting his body as at once scapegoat and helper. In the same letter he refers to "die Wunde, deren Sinnbild nur die Lungenwunde ist" (the wound of which the wound on my lungs is only a symbol). His life consists of "Jammer, Jammer" (woe and more woe) that cannot be "aufgeknotet" (unknotted). Tuberculosis is an infectious disease, not a conversion disorder, although Alexander subsumed it under the psychosomatic on the grounds that liability to infection is increased by the lowering of the immune system concomitant to distress.[10]

But granted that mind and body are reciprocally involved, is it the mind that is betraying the body, or vice versa? Everything hinges on the senses of "betray." According to the *Oxford English Dictionary*, it can denote "to play the part of traitor, to act treacherously"; or "to reveal (a secret) improperly or inadvertently"; or "to reveal one's true self, let out one's secret unconsciously." All these meanings are apposite to conversion disorders. The mind betrays the body, acting treacherously by resorting to the body to out psychological distress. It thereby indadvertently or unconsciously divulges a secret that becomes visible, as Freud put it, to those with eyes to see and ears to hear: "aus allen Poren dringt ihm der Verrat" (betrayal oozes out of him at every pore), for no mortal can keep a secret.[11] He or she cannot do so because the mind speaks involuntarily through the body. The circle of (self-)betrayal is completed in that the body betrays the mind into believing that the complaint is a somatic disease. The secret of the conversion disorder is "whispered everywhere," to use Congreve's words, in the literary work's metaphoricity.

Notes

PREFACE

1. "Somatization Disorder occurs only rarely in men in the United States," *DSM-IV*, 447; "Women with somatization disorder outnumber men 5 to 20 times, although the highest estimates may be due to the tendency not to diagnose somatization in male patients." *Synopsis of Psychiatry*, 617.
2. Weintraub, *Hysterical Conversion and Reactions* provides a list of some hundred pages of the tests to be performed on various organ systems before a diagnosis of a somatoform disorder can safely be made.
3. Kaplan et al., *Synopsis of Psychiatry*, 621.
4. Barbour, *Caring for Patients*, 3.
5. Lipowski, *Psychosomatic Medicine*, 112.
6. Dunbar, *Emotions and Bodily Changes*, xi.
7. Sontag, *Illness as Metaphor*, 21.
8. Charon, "The Great Empty Cup."

1. SPEAKING THROUGH THE BODY

1. Engel, "The Biopsychosocial Model and the Education of Health Professionals," 170.
2. *DSM-IV*, 462.
3. In an experiment at the Tavistock Clinic, London in the 1950s, the Hungaro-British psychiatrist Michael Balint trained family practitioners to listen to their patients' life problems as one way of alleviating their physical symptoms. See Balint, *The Doctor, the Patient, and His Illness*.
4. *DSM-IV*, 450; "employed" suggests a degree of conscious intentionality that generally does not come into play in psychosomatic disorders—in

201

contrast to malingering, where a tactic is more consciously "employed" for secondary gain.

5. Lipowski, *Psychosomatic Medicine*, 25.
6. Kaplan, Sadock, and Gelb, eds., *Synopsis of Psychiatry*, 619.
7. Halgin and Whitbourne, *Abnormal Psychology*, 239.
8. Sontag, *Illness as Metaphor*, 43.
9. Wolman, *Psychosomatic Disorders*, 23.
10. Marshall, review of Howard I. Kushner, *A Cursing Brain?*
11. See preface, note 1.
12. Lipowski, *Psychosomatic Medicine*, 25.
13. Alexander, *Psychosomatic Medicine*, 20.
14. Wolman, *Psychosomatic Disorders*, 55.
15. Dubovsky, *Mind-Body Deceptions*, 47.
16. Weiner, "Psychological Factors in Bodily Diseases," 31.
17. Sontag, *Illness as Metaphor*, 52–53.
18. Lipowski, *Psychosomatic Medicine*, 113.
19. Barbour, *Caring for Patients*, 38.
20. Janet, "Kyste parasitaire."
21. Alexander, *Psychosomatic Medicine*, 28.
22. Sontag, *Illness as Metaphor*, 54.
23. Theorell, Blomkvist, Lindh, and Evergard, "Cultural Life Events, Infections, and Symptoms During the Year Preceding Chronic Fatigue Syndrome."
24. Originally published in the journal *Psychosomatic Medicine* 46, no. 2 (1984): 153–71; reprinted in the collection *Psychosomatic Medicine*, 119–37.
25. Lipowski, *Psychosomatic Medicine*, 4.
26. Wolman, *Psychosomatic Disorders*, 7 and 3 respectively.
27. Lipowski, *Psychosomatic Medicine*, 13.
28. In considering alternatives to its present name, the American Psychosomatic Society has included as one of its options "Society for Biopsychosocial Medicine."
29. Engel, "The Biopsychosocial Model and Family Medicine," 409.
30. Sapira, "The Whole Patient Is Not Less Than the Sum of His Parts," 385.

2. SWINGS OF THE HISTORICAL PENDULUM

1. Rosenberg, "Body and Mind," 77.
2. Akerknecht, *Short History of Medicine*, 235.

3. Rosenberg, "Body and Mind," 77.
4. Akerknecht, *A Short History*, 235.
5. Jewson, "The Disappearance of the Sick Man," 228.
6. Cabanis, *Oeuvres philosophiques*, 2: 247.
7. Rush, *Sixteen Introductory Lectures*, 26.
8. Leake, ed., *Percival's Medical Ethics*, 222–23.
9. Léonard, *La France médicale*, 127.
10. See Schiller, "A Case of Brain Fever."
11. Later nineteenth-century cases include Edith in Anne Eliot's *Dr. Edith Romney* (1883), Jeanne in Maupassant's *Une Vie* (1883), Philip in Conan Doyle's "The Naval Treaty" (1884), and Jonathan Harker in Bram Stoker's *Dracula* (1897).
12. See Peterson, "Brain Fever in Nineteenth-Century Literature."
13. Alexander, *Psychosomatic Medicine*, 71.
14. Brontë, *Shirley*, 460.
15. Tatar, *Spellbound*, 5.
16. For further discussion of Mesmer see chapter 10 on *The Strange Case of Mademoiselle P.*
17. Warner, *Therapeutic Perspective*, 7.
18. Winter, *Mesmerized*, 4.
19. See Nuland, *Doctors*, 206–37, for a vivid evocation of Laënnec and the story of his invention.
20. Magnifying lenses had been used certainly since at least the sixteenth century, but the spherical shape of the lenses and their tendency to disperse ordinary light into the various colors of the spectrum resulted in visual aberrations that severely reduced their efficacy as a scientific tool. The greater their magnifying power, the greater proportionately also was their liability to distortion. This optical obstacle was removed in 1829 by Joseph Jackson Lister (1786–1869) with his achromatic microscope.
21. The practical possibilities of the improved microscope were quickly harnessed; by 1843, for example, the microscopic department at Guy's Hospital in London was examining phlegm from lungs, blood, urine, and mother's milk, and two years later instruction in its use was incorporated into the medical school curriculum.
22. See Furst, *Medical Progress*, 9.
23. Porter, *The Greatest Benefit*, 307.
24. Rosenberg, "Body and Mind," 84–85.
25. Ibid., 87.
26. Rather, *Medicine in the Eighteenth Century*, 15.
27. Rosenberg, "Body and Mind," 87.

28. Akerknecht, *Short History*, 205.
29. Drinka, *Birth of Neurosis*, 67-69.
30. Harrington, *Medicine, Mind, and the Double Brain*, 17–19.
31. Ibid., 177.
32. For differences in national traditions see Bynum, "The Nervous Patient in Eighteenth- and Nineteenth-Century Britain," 89–90.
33. Beard, *A Practical Treatise*, 36–117, and *American Nervousness*, 7–8.
34. Oppenheim, *"Shattered Nerves,"* 53.
35. For the spread of neurasthenia see Gosling, *Before Freud*, 32 and table 1, for patient occupations in the 217 cases surveyed.
36. Beard, *A Practical Treatise*, 8.
37. Beard, *American Nervousness*, 110–11.
38. Cleaves, *Autobiography of a Neurasthene*, 63; see also Furst, "'You Have Sprained Your Brain.'"
39. Goldstein, *Console and Classify*, 53.
40. "Nervous" was far preferable to "mental," which implied degeneracy or moral shortcomings. The distinction is clear in German in the difference between "Geisteskrankheiten" (diseases of the mind) and "Nervenkrankheiten" (diseases of the nervous system).
41. Drinka, *Birth of Neurosis*, 125.
42. Charcot, *L'Hystérie*, 70.
43. Ibid., 95.
44. Hodgkiss, "Chronic Pain"; Schivelbusch, *The Railway Journey*.
45. Furst, "Daniel Hack Tuke Walking a Tight-rope."
46. Freud, *Bruchstück einer Hysterie-Analyse; Fragment of an Analysis of a Case of Hysteria*.
47. Freud, *Gesammelte Werke* 1:108; *Standard Edition* 2:56.
48. Ellenberger, *Discovery of the Unconscious*.
49. Freud, *Ich und Es*, in *Gesammelte Werke*, 13:251; *Ego and Id*, in *Standard Edition* 19:12. Groddeck, *Das Buch vom Es*.
50. Deutsch, *Mysterious Leap*, 8.
51. Roazen, *Freud and His Followers*, 491.
52. Lipowski, *Psychosomatic Medicine*, 131.
53. In Deutsch, *Mysterious Leap*, 27–46.
54. Freud, *Gesammelte Werke*, 8:100; *Collected Papers*, 110–11.
55. Freud, *Gesammelte Werke*, 1:233.
56. Freud, *Gesammelte Werke*, 1:247.
57. Freud, *Gesammelte Werke*, 1:247.
58. Freud, *Gesammelte Werke*, 5:200.
59. Freud, *Gesammelte Werke*, 5:200; *Dora*, 57.
60. Freud, *Gesammelte Werke*, 5:213; *Dora*, 70–71.
61. Freud, *Gesammelte Werke*, 5:176; *Dora*, 32.

3. THE MYSTERIOUS LEAP

1. Freud, *Gesammelte Werke,* 11:265.
2. Freud, *General Introduction to Psychoanalysis,* 222.
3. Deutsch, *Mysterious Leap,* 9.
4. Halgin and Whitbourne, *Abnormal Psychology,* 247.
5. Rosenberg, "Body and Mind," 88.
6. *Psychosomatic Medicine,* 1:3.
7. An extensive correspondence between them remains unpublished.
8. Alexander, "Functional Disturbances of Psychogenic Nature," and "The Influence of Psychologic Factors Upon Gastrointestinal Disturbances."
9. Peabody, "Care of Patients," 878.
10. Shorter, *History of Psychiatry,* 302.
11. Luhrmann, *Of Two Minds,* 227.
12. See Shorter, *History of Psychiatry,* 298–305, and Young, *Harmony of Illusions,* 94–101.
13. Nemiah, "A Psychodynamic View of Psychosomatic Medicine," 299.
14. Storr, *Art of Psychotherapy,* 13.
15. Kutchins and Kirk, *Making Us Crazy,* 37.
16. Ibid., 21–54.
17. See Luhrmann, *Of Two Minds.*
18. Grinker, "'Open-system' Psychiatry," 115.
19. Merritt's *Textbook of Neurology,* 631 and 633. For a history of the understanding of epilepsy see Rice, *Dostoevsky and the Healing Arts.*
20. Levenstein, "The Very Model of a Modern Etiology."
21. Sapolsky, *Why Zebras Don't Get Ulcers.*
22. Asaad, *Psychosomatic Disorders,* 130.

4. LITERARY PATIENTS

1. Storr, *Churchill's Black Dog,* 3.
2. Freud, *Gesammelte Werke,* 8:240.
3. Freud, *Three Case Histories,* 104.
4. See Leo Bersani, *A Future for Astyanax: Character and Desire in Literature* (Boston: Little, Brown, 1976), and Peter Brooks, *Reading for the Plot* (New York: Vintage, 1984).
5. Lunbeck in *The Psychiatric Persuasion* shows how psychiatry changed toward the end of the nineteenth century "from a discipline primarily concerned with insanity to one equally concerned with normality, as focused on normal persons and their problems: sex, marriage,

womanhood and manhood, work, ambition, worldly failure, habits, desires, inclinations" (3).

6. Coleridge, *Biographia Literaria*, 2:6.
7. Furst, "Let's Pretend . . . ," *All Is True*, 28–47.
8. Even where the models are known, as in Flaubert's *Madame Bovary*, where Emma follows the pattern of two women, Mme. Delamare, and Mme. Pradier, Flaubert emphasized the typicality of her predicament in his comment that thousands of Emmas were weeping in the towns and villages of France.
9. Peterson, "Brain Fever in Nineteenth-Century Literature," 457.
10. Scott, *Bride of Lammermoor*, 238.
11. For another example see Balzac's *Le Lys das la vallée* (1833) for an understanding of the family dynamics of anorexia that anticipates medical writing by some forty years.
12. Brontë, *Wuthering Heights*, 10.
13. Maude Ellman, introduction to *Dracula*, viii.
14. *The Illustrated Sherlock Holmes Treasury*, 299.
15. Maupassant, *Une Vie*, 111.
16. Barbour, *Caring for Patients*, 191.
17. Lipowski, *Psychosomatic Medicine*, 132.
18. Ibid., 112 and 33.
19. Storr, *Art of Psychotherapy*, 3.
20. Lipowski, *Psychosomatic Medicine*, 33–35.
21. Alexander, *Psychosomatic Medicine*, 46.
22. Kleinman, *Illness Narratives*, 182.
23. Kaplan, Sadock, and Grebb, *Synopsis of Psychiatry*, 620.
24. Alexander, *Psychosomatic Medicine*, 264.
25. Lipowski, *Psychosomatic Medicine*, 11.
26. Wolman, *Psychosomatic Medicine*, 48.
27. Deutsch, *Mysterious Leap*, 77.
28. Barbour, *Caring for Patients*, 119.
29. Kaplan, Sadock, and Grebb, *Synopsis of Psychiatry*, 621.
30. Alexander, *Psychosomatic Medicine*, 42.
31. This previously predominant understanding of the conversion symptom as a symbol has only recently been subjected to serious questioning by psychopharmacologists, who argue against any direct psychological association between a putative secret and a manifest symptom; instead they focus on brain chemistry and physiological processes.
32. Ellenberger, *Discovery of the Unconscious*, 46.
33. Ibid., 43–44.

34. Freud, *Gesammelte Werke*, 5:197; *Dora*, 54. "Conceals" suggests too deliberate an action; the German "deckt" (literally: "covers") is rather more open, and perhaps passive.
35. Ibid., 5:198, and 56 respectively.
36. Cited in Bok, *Secrets*, 8, from Carl Jung.
37. See Jackson, "The Talking Cures," in *Care of the Psyche*, 98–113.

5. "A STRANGE SYMPATHY BETWIXT SOUL AND BODY"

1. Lipowski, *Psychosomatic Medicine*, 132.
2. Delbanco, *Puritan Ordeal*, 218.
3. Erikson, *Wayward Puritans*, 72
4. "You are the light of the world. A city that is set on a hill cannot be hid." *Matthew* 5:14.
5. John Davenport, *A Profession of faith made at his admission into the Churches of God;* quoted in Bremer, *Shaping New Englands*, 10.
6. Bremer, *Shaping New Englands*, 42
7. Delbanco, *Puritan Ordeal*, 3
8. *DSM-IV*, 451.
9. Heimert and Delbanco, *Puritans in America*, 14–15
10. Ellenberger, *Discovery of the Unconscious*, 45.
11. Erikson, *Wayward Puritans*, 73
12. Delbanco, *Puritan Ordeal*, 97
13. Bremer, *Shaping New Englands*, 49.
14. Delbanco, *Puritan Ordeal*, 221.

6. NERVES: AT THE INTERSTICES OF PHYSIOLOGY AND PSYCHOLOGY

1. *Century of Struggle*, 76. My thanks to Edith Gelles for this citation.
2. Tuke, *Influence of the Mind Upon the Body*, xii.
3. See pp. 30–31.
4. Drinka, *Birth of Neurosis*, 29–30.
5. See pp. 28–29.
6. Freud's *Studies on Hysteria* appeared in 1895.
7. Only ten years before, Flaubert had been indicted for "offenses à la morale publique et à la religion" for his quite discreet treatment of adultery by a middle-class woman in *Madame Bovary* (1857).
8. Zola, *Une Campagne*, 129.

9. Zola, *Thérèse Raquin,* 24.
10. Although hysteria was commonly associated with women, it was known also to affect men. See Briquet, *Traité clinique et thérapeutique de l'hystérie,* 51; and Micale, "Charcot and the Idea of Hysteria in the Male."

7. "A SICK SPOT ON THE BODY OF THE FAMILY"

1. Mann, *Buddenbrooks,* 272; all translations are by Lilian R. Furst.
2. For a fine overview of the historical situation see Ridley, *Mann: Buddenbrooks,* 10–19; also Beaton, "Die Zeitgeschichte," in *Buddenbrooks-Handbuch,* ed. Moulden and Wilpert, 201–11.
3. Lipowski, *Psychosomatic Medicine,* 132.
4. See, Wilpert, "Das Bild der Gesellschaft" in *Buddenbrooks-Handbuch,* ed. Moulden and Wilpert, 244–58.
5. Sagave, "Zur Geschichtlichkeit von Thomas Manns Jugendroman."
6. *DSM-IV,* 446.
7. Ibid., 457.
8. Ibid., 447.
9. Alexander, *Psychosomatic Medicine,* 264.
10. Moulden and Wilpert, *Buddenbrooks-Handbuch,* 21
11. Heller, *Ironic German,* 47.
12. Heilbut, *Thomas Mann,* 98.
13. *DSM-IV,* 447.
14. Heilbut, *Thomas Mann,* 98
15. Ibid., 100.
16. Ibid., 102
17. One-third to one-half of patients initially diagnosed with a somatoform disorder turn out eventually to have a verifiable disease (*DSM-IV,* 453).
18. Ridley, *Thomas Mann: "Buddenbrooks,"* 33.

8. "LEGS TURNED TO BUTTER"

1. For "Diagnostic Criteria for Conversion Disorder" see chapter 1:7.
2. *DSM-IV,* 454.
3. Dinnerstein, "Antisemitism," 212.
4. Ibid., 212.
5. Scholnick, *The New Deal,* 65–73.
6. Lipowski, *Psychosomatic Medicine,* 132.
7. Barbour, *Caring for Patients,* 193.
8. Lipowski, *Psychosomatic Medicine,* 35.

9. Deutsch, *Mysterious Leap,* 45.
10. E.g., Alexander, *Psychosomatic Medicine,* 142–63; Asaad, *Psychosomatic Disorders,* 77–82; Dubovsky, *Mind-Body Deceptions,* Dunbar, *Emotions and Bodily Changes,* 201–38, and *Psychosomatic Diagnosis,* 248–366; Wolman, *Psychosomatic Disorders,* 133–44.
11. I want to record my gratitude to Esther Zago for reading and discussing successive drafts of this chapter. Also to her student, Ashima Gupta, for permission to read her paper. Both made stimulating suggestions.

9. SUBSTANCE AND SHADOW

1. See Buranelli, *Wizard from Vienna,* 75–88; Ellenberger, *Discovery of the Unconscious,* 57–69; Tatar, *Spellbound,* 3–25.
2. Lipowski, *Psychosomatic Medicine,* 132.
3. Buranelli, *Wizard from Vienna,* 85.
4. Freud's patient, Cäcilie, in his *Studies on Hysteria,* experiences a comment by her husband as a slap in the face that is subsequently converted into recurrent attacks of facial neuralgia.
5. See Ellenberger, *Discovery of the Unconscious,* 70–83; Tatar, *Spellbound,* 6, 35–44.

10. SHELL SHOCK

1. Young, *Harmony of Illusions,* 50
2. See Schivelbusch, *The Railway Journey,* 135–45.
3. Goldstein, "The Uses of Male Hysteria;" Micale, "Charcot and the Idea of Hysteria in the Male."
4. Leed, *No Man's Land,* 166.
5. Ibid., 166.
6. (London, 1931), 255.
7. Leed, *No Man's Land,* 185.
8. *DSM-IV,* 429
9. Ferguson, *Pity of War,* 341.
10. *Report of the War Office Committee of Enquiry into "Shell Shock"* (London, 1922), 57–58; cited by Leed, *No Man's Land,* 182.
11. The publication of Barker's trilogy (*Regeneration* was followed by *The Eye in the Door* [1993] and *The Ghost Road* [1995], which was awarded Britain's premier literary prize, the Booker) certainly contributed to the recent renewal of his fame. An article in *The Lancet* of 19 July 1997

by Katherine G. Nickerson and Steven Shea, "W. H. R. Rivers: Portrait of a Great Physician in Pat Barker's *Regeneration* Trilogy," is a direct outcome of the novels.

12. Rivers, "The Repression of War Experience," 174.
13. For a summary of the fundamental differences between Rivers and Freud see Young, *Harmony of Illusions*, 77.
14. Rivers, *Conflict and Dream*, 144.
15. Cited in Leed, *No Man's Land*, 176–77.
16. See Renoir's 1938 film *La Grande Illusion*.
17. Leed, *No Man's Land*, 118
18. In January 1918, Noel Pemberton Billing, a demagogic, extreme right-wing member of the British parliament, claimed the existence of a "Black Book" listing the names of Britons who had been corrupted by the German, including 47,000 "perverts." Reference to the rumors about this document in *Regeneration* represents another crossover of fact into fiction.
19. Rivers, *Con flict and Dream*, 166.
20. Barker, *The Ghost Road*, 274.

11. OUTING THE DISTRESS

1. Dostoevsky, *The Idiot*, 167.
2. Sapira, "The Whole Patient," 385.
3. Nemiah, "A Psychodynamic View," 299 and 301.
4. Freud, *Gesammelte Werke*, 1:227; *Standard Edition*, 2:160.
5. Sacks, *Man Who Mistook His Wife for a Hat*, 183.
6. Ibid., 178.
7. Freud, "Psychogene Sehstörung," 97; "Psychogenic Visual Disturbance," 107.
8. Sontag, *Illness as Metaphor*, 39.
9. Kafka, *Briefe*, 161.
10. Alexander, *Psychosomatic Medicine*, 51.
11. Freud, *Bruchstück einer Hysterie-Analyse*, 240; *Dora*, 120.

Bibliography

PRIMARY SOURCES

Alexander, Franz. "Functional Disturbances of a Psychogenic Nature." *Journal of the American Medical Association* 100 (18 February 1933): 469–73.

———. *Psychosomatic Medicine: Its Principles and Applications.* New York: W. W. Norton, 1950.

———. "The Influence of Psychologic Factors upon Gastrointestinal Disturbances." *Psychoanalytic Quarterly* 3 (1934): 501–39.

Balzac, Honoré de. *Le Cousin Pons.* 1847. Reprint, Paris: Gallimard, 1963.

Banville, John. *The Untouchable.* (1997) New York: Vintage International, 1998.

Barbour, Allen B. *Caring for Patients: A Critique of the Medical Model.* Stanford: Stanford University Press, 1995.

Barker, Pat. *Regeneration.* 1991. New York: Plume, 1993.

———. *The Eye in the Door.* 1993. New York: Plume, 1995.

———. *The Ghost Road.* 1995. New York: Dutton, 1995.

Beard, George M. *American Nervousness: Its Causes and Consequences.* New York: Putnam's, 1881.

———. *A Practical Treatise on Nervous Exhaustion (Neurasthenia).* 1881. 5th ed. enlarged and edited by A. P. Rockwell. Reprint, New York: Kraus, 1971.

———. "The Influence of the Mind in the Causation and Cure of Disease—The Potency of Definite Expectations." *Journal of Nervous and Mental Diseases* 4 (1877): 429–34.

———. "Neurasthenia or Nervous Exhaustion." *Boston Medical and Surgical Journal* 80 (1869): 217–22.

Briquet, Pierre. *Traité clinique et thérapeutique de l'hystérie.* Paris: J.-B. Baillière et Fils, 1859.

Brontë, Charlotte. *Shirley.* 1849. Reprint, New York: Dutton, 1965.

Brontë, Emily. *Wuthering Heights.* 1847. Reprint, New York: NAL, 1959.

Cabanis, Pierre Jean Georges. *Oeuvres philosophiques.* 2 vols. Paris: Presses universitaires de France, 1956.

Carr, Caleb. *The Angel of Darkness.* 1997. New York: Ballantine Books, 1998.

Charcot, Jean-Martin. *L'Hystérie.* Textes choisis et présentés par E. Trillat. Toulouse: Privat, 1971.

Cleaves, Margaret. *The Autobiography of a Neurasthene.* Boston: Graham Press, 1910.

Coleridge, Samuel Taylor. *Biographia Literaria.* 2 vols. 1817. New ed. by James Engell and Walter Jackson Bate. Princeton: Princeton University Press, 1983.

Corp, William. *Essay on the Changes Produced in the Body by Operations of the Mind.* London: Ridgway, 1791.

Dickens, Charles. *Great Expectations.* 1860. Reprint, New York: Oxford University Press, 1994.

Doyle, Arthur Conan. "Naval Treaty." 1892. Reprinted in *The Illustrated Sherlock Holmes Treasury,* 292–313. New York: Avenel, 1984.

———. "Copper Beeches." 1892. Reprinted in *The Illustrated Sherlock Holmes Treasury,* 156–71. New York: Avenel, 1984.

Dostoevsky, Fyodor. *The Brothers Karamazov.* 1866. Reprint, New York: Norton, 1976.

———. *The Idiot.* 1860. Translated by Alan Myers. New York: Oxford University Press, 1992.

DSM (Diagnostic and Statistical Manual of the American Psychiatric Association). vol. I, 1952; vol II, 1968; vol III, 1980; vol IV, edited by Allen Francis, 1994. Washington: American Psychiatric Association.

Dunbar, H. Flanders. *Emotions and Bodily Changes: A Survey of Literature on Psychosomatic Interrelationships, 1910–1933.* 1935. 2d. rev. ed., New York: Columbia University Press, 1938.

———. *Psychosomatic Diagnosis.* 1943. 2d. ed., New York: Paul B. Hoeber, 1948.

Eliot, Anne. *Dr. Edith Romney.* London: Richard Bentley & Son, 1883.

Engel, George L. "The Biopsychosocial Model and the Education of Health Professionals." *Annals of the New York Academy of Sciences* 310 (1978): 169–81.

———. "The Biopsychosocial Model and Family Medicine." *Journal of Family Practice* 16, no. 2 (1983): 409–13.

———. "The Clinical Application of the Biopsychosocial Model." *American Journal of Psychiatry* 137, no. 5 (May 1980): 535–44.

————. "The Need for a New Medical Model: A Challenge for Biomedicine." *Science* 196 (8 April 1977): 129–36.

Falconer, William. *Dissertation on the Influence of the Passions upon Disorders of the Body.* London: Dilly, 1796.

Flaubert, Gustave, *Madame Bovary.* 1857. Reprint, Paris: Gallimard, 1947. English ed. translated and edited by Paul de Man. New York: W. W. Norton, 1965.

Freud, Sigmund. *Bruchstück einer Hysterie-Analyse.* 1905. Reprinted in *Gesammelte Werke,* vol. 5 (1904–5), 161–286 London: Imago, 1942. English translation, *Dora: An Analysis of a Case of Hysteria.* New York: Collier, 1963.

————. *Complete Letters of Sigmund Freud to Wilhelm Fliess, 1887–1904,* translated and edited by Jeffrey Moussaieff Masson. Cambridge, Mass.: Harvard University Press, 1985. Original German edition, *Sigmund Freud Briefe an Wilhelm Fliess,* edited by Michael Schröter. Frankfurt: Fischer, 1986.

————. *Das Ich und das Es.* 1923. Reprinted in *Gesammelte Werke,* vol. 13 (1920–24), 239–89 London: Imago, 1940. English translation, *The Ego and the Id,* in *Standard Edition,* translated and edited by John Strachey, 3–66. New York: Norton 1961.

————. "Die psychogene Sehstörung in psychoanalytischer Auffassung." 1910. Reprinted in *Gesammelte Werke,* vol. 8 (1909–13), 94–102 [1943]; London: Imago, 1948. English translation "Psychogenic Visual Disturbance According to Psychoanalytical Conceptions." in *Collected Papers,* translated by Joan Riviere, 2: 105–12 London: Hogarth, 1953.

————. "Psychoanalytische Bemerkungen über einen autobiographisch beschriebenen Fall von Paranoia (Dementia Paranoides)." 1911. Reprinted in *Gesammelte Werke,* vol. 8 (1909–13), 239–320 London: Imago, 1943. English translation, "Psychoanalytic Notes upon an Autobiographical Account of a Case of Paranoia (Dementia Paranoides)," in *Three Case Histories,* 103–86 New York: Collier Books, 1963.

————. *Studien über Hysterie.* 1895. Reprinted in *Gesammelte Werke,* vol. 1 (1892–95), 75–251 London: Imago, 1952 English translation, *Studies on Hysteria* in *Standard Edition,* vol. 2, translated and edited by John Strachey (1961).

————. *Vorlesungen zur Einführung in die Psychoanalyse.* Reprinted in *Gesammelte Werke,* vol. 11 (1916–17) [1944]; 7th ed., London: Imago, 1978. English translation, *A General Introduction to Psychoanalysis.* [1920]; 16th ed., New York: Boni & Liveright, 1926.

Gaskell, Elizabeth. *Ruth.* 1853. Reprint, New York: Oxford University Press, 1998.

————. *Wives and Daughters.* 1866. Reprint, New York: Penguin, 1969.

Groddeck, Georg. *Das Buch vom Es.* Leipzig: Internationaler Psychoanalytischer Verlag, 1923.

Hawthorne, Nathaniel. *The Scarlet Letter.* 1850. Reprint, New York: Signet, 1959.

Holmes, Oliver Wendell. *Elsie Venner.* 1861. Reprint, Boston: Houghton Mifflin, 1886.

James, Henry. *The Wings of the Dove.* 1902. Reprint, New York: Dell, 1962.

Janet, Pierre. "Les Actes inconscients et le dédoublement de la personnalité pendant le somnambulisme provoqué." *Revue philosophique* 22 (1886): 577–92.

————. "Etude sur un cas d'amnésie antérograde dans la maladie de la désagrégation psychologique." In *International Congress of Experimental Psychology,* 26–30. London: Williams & Norgate, 1892.

————. "Kyste parasitaire du cerveau." *Archives générales de médecine* 28, no. 2 (1891): 464–72.

Kafka, Franz. *Briefe, 1902–1924.* New York: Schocken Books, 1958.

Harold Kaplan, Benjamin Sadock, and Jack Grebb, eds. *Synopsis of Psychiatry,* 7th ed. Baltimore: Williams & Wilkins, 1994.

Leake, Chauncey D., ed. *Percival's Medical Ethics.* Baltimore: Williams & Wilkins, 1927.

Léonard, Jacques. *La France médicale au XIXe siècle.* Paris: Juillard, 1978.

Lipowski, Zbigniew J. *Psychosomatic Medicine and Liaison Psychiatry: Selected Papers.* New York: Plenum, 1985.

Mann, Thomas. *Buddenbrooks.* 1900. Reprint, Frankfurt: Fischer, 1961. English translation by John Woods. New York: Knopf, 1993.

Maupassant, Guy de. *Pierre et Jean.* 1887. Reprint, Paris: Albin Michel, 1968. English translation by Martin Turnell London: New English Library, 1962.

————. *Une vie.* 1883. Reprint, Paris: Albin Michel, 1970. English translation, *A Woman's Life,* translated by H. H. P. Sloman. Harmondsworth: Penguin [1965], 1967.

Miller, Arthur. *Broken Glass.* New York: Penguin, 1994.

Mitchell, Silas Weir. *Lectures on Diseases of the Nervous System.* Philadelphia: Henry C. Lea, 1885.

O'Connor, Flannery. "The Enduring Chill." 1956. Reprinted in *Complete Stories,* 109–39 New York: Farrar, Straus & Giroux, 1965.

O'Doherty, Brian. *The Strange Case of Mademoiselle P.* New York: Pantheon, 1992.

Rather, L. J. *Mind and Body in Eighteenth-Century Medicine: A Study Based on Jerome Gaub's "De regimine mentis."* Berkeley: University of California Press, 1965.

Rivers, W. H. R. *Conflict and Dream.* London: Kegan Paul, 1923.

———. "Freud's Psychology of the Unconscious." *Lancet* (16 June 1917): 912–14.

———. "The Repression of War Experience." *Lancet* (2 February 1918): 172–77.

Rush, Benjamin. *Sixteen Introductory Lectures.* Philadelphia: Bradford & Innskeep, 1811.

Scott, Walter. *The Bride of Lammermoor.* 1819. Reprinted in *The Waverley Novels,* edited by J. H. Alexander, vol. 7 New York: Columbia University Press, 1995.

Stoker, Bram. *Dracula.* 1897. Reprint, New York: Oxford University Press, 1996.

Thorell, Blomquist, Lingh, and Everhard. "Cultural Life Events, Infections, and Symptoms During the Year Preceding Chronic Fatigue Syndrome." *Psychosomatic Medicine* 54, no. 3 (March-April 1992): 231–46.

Tuke, Daniel Hack. *Illustrations of the Influence of the Mind Upon the Body in Health and Disease.* 1872. 2d ed., Philadelphia: Henry C. Lea, 1884.

Weiss, Edward, and O. Spurgeon English. *Psychosomatic Medicine: The Clinical Application of Psychopathology to General Medical Problems.* Philadelphia: Saunders, 1943.

Yealland, Lewis. *Hysterical Disorders of Warfare.* London: Macmillan, 1918.

Zola, Emile. *Thérèse Raquin.* 1866. Reprint, Paris: Fasquelle, 1968. English translation by L. W. Tancock, Harmondsworth: Penguin, 1962.

———. *Une Campagne.* 1880–81. Reprint, Paris: Charpentier, 1913.

SECONDARY SOURCES

Abse, D. Wilfred. *Hysteria and Related Mental Disorders.* Bristol: Wright, 1987.

Adler, R. and Cohen, N. "Behavior and the Immune System." In *Handbook of Behavioral Medicine,* ed. W. D. Gentry, 117–73 New York: Guilford Press, 1984.

Akerknecht, Erwin. *A Short History of Medicine.* 1955. 2d rev. ed., Baltimore: Johns Hopkins University Press, 1982.

Asaad, Ghazi. *Psychosomatic Disorders: Theoretical and Clinical Aspects.* New York: Brunner/Mazel, 1996.

Balint, Michael. *The Doctor, the Patient, and His Illness.* New York: International Press, 1957.

Beaton, Kenneth B. "Die Zeitgeschichte und ihre Integrierung im Roman." In *Buddenbrooks-Handbuch,* edited by Ken Moulden and Gero von Wilpert, 201–11. Stuttgart: Alfred Körner, 1988.

Beizer, Janet. *Ventriloqized Bodies: Narratives of Hysteria in Nineteenth-Century France.* Ithaca: Cornell Univ. Press, 1998.

Berrios, German E., and Roy Porter, eds. *A History of Clinical Psychiatry: The Origin and History of Psychiatric Disorders.* New York: New York University Press, 1985.

Blustein, Bonnie Ellen. "'A Hollow Square of Psychological Science': American Neurologists and Psychologists in Conflict." In *Madhouses, Mad-Doctors, and Madmen: The Social History of Psychiatry in the Victorian Era,* edited by Andrew Scull, 241–70 Philadelphia: University of Pennsylvania Press, 1981.

Bok, Sissela. *Secrets: On the Ethics of Concealment and Revelation.* [1983.] New York: Vintage, 1989.

Brady, Patrick. "Body and Brain, Mind and Soul." *Synthesis* 2, no. 2 (fall 1997): 5–15.

Bremer, Francis J. *Shaping New Englands: Puritan Clergymen in Seventeenth-Century England and New England.* New York: Twayne, 1994.

Buranelli, Vincent. *The Wizard from Vienna.* New York: Coward, McCann & Geoghan, 1975.

Bynum, W. F. "The Nervous Patient in Eighteenth- and Nineteenth-Century Britain: The Psychiatric Origins of British Neurology." In *The Anatomy of Madness,* edited by W. F. Bynum, R. Porter, and M. Shepherd, 1:89–102 New York: Routledge, 1985.

Charon, Rita. "The Great Empty Cup of Attention: The Doctor and the Illness in *The Wings of the Dove.*" *Literature and Medicine* 9 (1990): 105–24.

Delbanco, Andrew. *The Puritan Ordeal.* Cambridge, Mass.: Harvard University Press, 1989.

Deutsch, Felix. *On the Mysterious Leap from the Mind to the Body.* New York: International University Press, 1959.

Dinnerstein, Leonard. "Antisemitism in Crisis Times in the United States: The 1920s and 1930s." In *Anti-Semitism in Times of Crisis,* edited by Sander L. Gilman and Steven T. Katz, 212–26 New York: New York University Press, 1991.

Drinka, George F. *The Birth of Neurosis: Myth, Malady and the Victorians.* New York: Simon & Schuster, 1984.

Dubovsky, Steven L. *Mind-Body Deceptions: The Psychosomatics of Everyday Life.* New York: W. W. Norton, 1997.

Ellenberger, Henri F. *The Discovery of the Unconscious: The History and Evolution of Dynamic Psychotherapy.* New York: Basic Books, 1980.

———. "The Pathogenic Secret and Its Therapeutics." *Journal of the History of the Behavioral Sciences* 2 (1966): 29–42.

Erikson, Kai T. *Wayward Puritans: A Study in the Sociology of Deviance.* New York: John Wiley & Sons, 1966.

Ey, Henri. "History and Analysis of the Concept of Hysteria." *La Revue du practicien* 14 (1964): 1417–34. Reprinted in *Hysteria*, edited by Alec Roy, 1–16 New York: John Wiley & Sons, 1982.

Ferguson, Niall. *The Pity of War*. New York: Basic Books, 1999.

Flexner, Eleanor. *Century of Struggle: The Women's Rights Movement in the United States*. Cambridge, Mass.: Harvard University Press, 1959.

Furst, Lilian R. *All Is True: The Claims and Strategies of Realist Fiction*. Durham, N.C.: Duke University Press, 1995.

———. "Anxious Patients/Anxious Doctor: Telling Stories in Freud's *Studies on Hysteria*." *LIT* 8 (1998): 259–77.

———. "Daniel Hack Tuke Walking a Tight-rope." *Nineteenth-Century Prose* 27, no. 1 (spring 2000): 60–74.

———. *Medical Progress and Social Reality: A Reader in Nineteenth-Century Medicine and Literature*. Albany: State University of New York Press, 2000.

———. "'You Have Sprained Your Brain': Margaret Cleaves's *Autobiography of a Neurasthene*." *Nineteenth-Century Prose* 25, no. 1 (spring 1998): 140–53.

Goldstein, Jan. *Console and Classify: The French Psychiatric Profession in the Nineteenth Century*. New York: Cambridge University Press, 1987.

———. "The Uses of Male Hysteria: Medical and Literary Discourse in Nineteenth-Century France." *Representations* 34 (1991): 134–65.

Gosling, F. G. *Before Freud: Neurasthenia and the American Medical Community, 1870–1910*. Urbana: University of Illinois Press, 1987.

Grinker, R. R. "'Open-system' Psychiatry." *American Journal of Psychoanalysis* 26 (1966): 110–17.

Halgin, Richard P., and Susan K. Whitbourne. *Abnormal Psychology: The Human Experience of Psychological Disorders*. Fort Worth, Tex.: Harcourt Brace Jovanovich, 1993.

Harrington, Anne. *Medicine and the Double Brain in Nineteenth-Century Thought*. Princeton, New Jersey: Princeton University Press, 1987.

Heilbut, Anthony. *Thomas Mann: Eros and Literature*. New York: Knopf, 1996.

Heimert, Alan, and Andrew Delbanco. *The Puritans in America: A Narrative Anthology*. Cambridge, Mass.: Harvard University Press, 1985.

Heller, Erich. *The Ironic German*. London: Secker & Warburg, 1958.

Hodgkiss, A.-D. "Chronic Pain in Nineteenth-Century British Medical Writings." *History of Psychiatry* 2, no. 5, pt. 1 (March 1991): 27–40.

Horowitz, Mardi J., ed. *Hysterical Personality*. New York: Jason Aronson, 1977.

Jackson, Stanley W. *Care of the Psyche*. New Haven: Yale University Press, 1999.

Jewson, N. D. "The Disappearance of the Sick Man from Medical Cosmology, 1770–1870." *Sociology* 10 (1976): 225–44.

Kleinman, Arthur. *The Illness Narratives: Suffering, Healing, and the Human Condition.* New York: Basic Books, 1988.

Krohn, Alan. *Hysteria: The Elusive Neurosis.* Psychological Issues 12, nos. 1–2, Monograph 45/6. New York: International University Press, 1978.

Kutchins, Herb, and Stuart A. Kirk. *Making Us Crazy: DSM, the Psychiatric Bible and the Creation of Mental Disorders.* New York: Free Press, 1997.

———. *The Selling of DSM: The Rhetoric of Science in Psychiatry.* Hawthorne, N.Y.: Aldine de Gruyter, 1992.

Leed, Eric J. *No Man's Land: Combat and Identity in World War I.* London: Cambridge University Press, 1979.

Levenstein, Susan. "The Very Model of a Modern Etiology: A Biopsychosocial View of Peptic Ulcer." *Psychosomatic Medicine* 62, no. 2 (March–April 2000): 176–85.

Luhrmann, T. M. *Of Two Minds: The Growing Disorder in American Psychiatry.* New York: Knopf, 2000.

Lunbeck, Elizabeth. *The Psychiatric Persuasion: Knowledge, Gender, and Power in Modern America.* Princeton: Princeton University Press, 1994.

Lutz, Tom. *American Nervousness, 1903: An Anecdotal History.* Ithaca: Cornell University Press, 1991.

Marshall, John C. Review of Howard I Kushner, *A Cursing Brain: The History of Tourette Syndrome. Times Literary Supplement,* 29 October 1999, 9.

Massonneu, Grace. "A Social Analysis of a Group of Psychoneurotic Ex-Servicemen." *Mental Hygiene* 6 (1922): 575–91.

Medical Meanings: A Glossary of Word Origins, edited William S. Haubrich. Philadelphia: American College of Physicians, 1997.

Merritt, Hiram Houston. *Textbook of Neurology.* Ed. Lewis P. Rowland. Philadelphia: Lea & Febinger, 1984.

Micale, Mark S. "Charcot and the Idea of Hysteria in the Male: Gender, Mental Science, and Medical Diagnosis in Late Nineteenth-Century France." *Medical History* 34 (1990): 363–411.

Moulden, Ken, and Gero von Wilpert, eds. *Buddenbrooks-Handbuch.* Stuttgart: Alfred Körner, 1988.

Nemiah, John C. "A Psychodynamic View of Psychosomatic Medicine." *Psychosomatic Medicine* 62, no. 3 (May–June 2000): 299–303.

Nickerson, Katherine G., and Steven Shea. "W. H. R. Rivers: Portrait of a Great Physician in Pat Barker's *Regeneration* Trilogy." *Lancet,* 350 (19 July 1997): 205–9.

Nuland, Sherwin B. *Doctors: The Biography of Medicine.* [1988.] New York: Vintage, 1989.

Oppenheim, Janet. *"Shattered Nerves": Doctors, Patients, and Depression in Victorian England.* New York: Oxford University Press, 1991.

Parsons, Talcott. *The Social System.* New York: Free Press, 1961.

Peabody, Frances W. "The Care of Patients." *Journal of the American Medical Association* 88, no. 2 (1927): 877–81.

Peterson, Audrey C. "Brain Fever in Nineteenth-Century Literature: Fact and Fiction." *Victorian Studies* 19 (June 1976): 445–64.

Porter, Roy. *The Greatest Benefit to Mankind: A Medical History of Humanity.* 1997. New York: W. W. Norton, 1998.

Reik, Theodor. *Listening with the Third Ear.* New York: Farrar, Straus, 1949.

Rice, James L. *Dostoevsky and the Healing Arts.* Ann Arbor: Ardis, 1985.

Ridley, Hugh. *Thomas Mann: Buddenbrooks.* London: Cambridge University Press, 1987.

Roazen, Paul. *Freud and His Followers.* New York: Knopf, 1971.

Rosenberg, Charles E. "Body and Mind in Nineteenth-Century Medicine." In *Explaining Epidemics and Other Studies in the History of Medicine,* 74–89 New York: Cambridge University Press, 1992.

———. "The Place of George M. Beard in Nineteenth-Century Psychiatry." *Bulletin of the History of Medicine* 36 (1962): 245–59.

Roy, Alec, ed. *Hysteria.* New York: John Wiley & Sons, 1982.

Sacks, Oliver. *An Anthropologist on Mars: Seven Paradoxical Tales.* New York, Knopf, 1995.

———. *The Man Who Mistook His Wife for a Hat and Other Stories.* [1970.] New York: Basic Books, 1986.

Sagave, Pierre-Paul. "Zur Geschichtlichkeit von Thomas Manns Jugendroman: Bürgerliches Klassenbewusstsein und kapitalistische Praxis in *Buddenbrooks.*" In *Literaturwissenschaft und Geschichtsphilosophie. Festschrift für Wilhelm Emrich,* 436–52. Berlin: Aufbau, 1975.

Sapira, Joseph D. "The Whole Patient Is Not Less Than the Sum of His Parts." *Psychosomatic Medicine* 54, no. 4 (July–August 1992): 383–93.

Sapolsky, Robert M. *Why Zebras Don't Get Heart Attacks: A Guide to Stress, Stress-Related Diseases, and Coping.* [1994.] New York: W. H. Freeman, 1998.

Schiller, Francis. "A Case of Brain Fever." *Clio Medica* 9, no. 3 (1974): 181–92.

Schivelbusch, Wolfgang. *Geschichte der Eisenbahn.* Munich: Carl Hanser, 1978. English translation, *The Railway Journey: Trains and Travel in the Nineteenth Century,* translated by Anselm Hollo New York: Urizen Books, 1979.

Scholnick, Myron L. *The New Deal and Anti-Semitism in America.* New York: Garland, 1990.

Scull, Andrew, ed. *Madhouses, Mad-Doctors, and Madmen: The Social History of Psychiatry in the Victorian Era.* Philadelphia: University of Pennsylvania Press, 1981.

Shorter, Edward. *A History of Psychiatry: From the Era of the Asylum to the Age of Prozac.* New York: Wiley, 1997.

————. *From Paralysis to Fatigue: A History of Psychosomatic Illness in the Modern Era*. New York: Free Press, 1992.

Showalter, Elaine. *The Female Malady: Women, Madness, and English Culture, 1830–1980*. New York: Penguin Books, 1985.

Slavney, Phillip R. *Perspectives on "Hysteria"*. Baltimore: Johns Hopkins University Press, 1990.

Sontag, Susan. *Illness as Metaphor*. [1977.] New York: Vintage, 1979.

Storr, Anthony. *The Art of Psychotherapy*. 1980. 2nd. rev. ed., New York: Routledge, 1990.

————. *Churchill's Black Dog, Kafka's Mice, and Other Phenomena of the Human Mind*. New York: Grove Press, 1988.

Tatar, Maria M. *Spellbound: Studies in Mesmerism and Literature*. Princeton: Princeton University Press, 1978.

Veith, Ilza. *Hysteria: The History of a Disease*. [1965.] Chicago: University of Chicago Press, 1970.

Walton, John, Jeremiah A. Barondess, and Stephen Lock, eds. *The Oxford Medical Companion*. New York: Oxford University Press, 1994.

Warner, John Harley, *The Therapeutic Perspective*. Cambridge, Mass.: Harvard University Press, 1986.

Weiner, H. "Psychological Factors in Bodily Diseases." In *Handbook of Clinical Health Psychology*, edited by T. Millon, C. Green, and R. Meagher, 31–52 New York: Plenum, 1982.

————. "Contemporary Research and the Mind/Body Problem." In *Body and Mind*, edited by R. W. Rieber, 223–40 New York: Academic Press, 1980.

Weintraub, Michael I. *Hysterical Conversion and Reactions: A Clinical Guide to Diagnosis and Treatment*. New York: SP Medical and Scientific Books, 1983.

Wilpert, Gero von. "Das Bild der Gesellschaft." In *Buddenbrooks-Handbuch*, ed. Ken Moulden and Gero von Wilpert, 245–58 Stuttgart: Alfred Körner, 1988.

Winter, Alison. *Mesmerized: Powers of Mind in Victorian Britain*. Chicago: University of Chicago Press, 1998.

Wise, T. N. "The Somatizing Patient." *Annals of Clinical Psychiatry* 4 (1992): 9–16.

Wolman, Benjamin B. *Psychosomatic Disorders*. New York: Plenum, 1988.

Young, Allan. *The Harmony of Illusions: Inventing Post-Traumatic Stress Disorder*. Princeton: Princeton University Press, 1995.

Index

suggestion, power of, 24, 33, 142, 166, 178
Sydenham, Thomas, 21
Synopsis of Psychiatry, 6, 8, 12, 66, 193

Talking cure, 61, 66, 68, 126, 142–43, 178, 184, 189, 196
See also psychotherapy
Textbook of Neurology, 11
Thérèse Raquin, 63, 93–109, 117, 195, 197, 198
See also Zola, Émile
Tuke, Daniel Hack, 30–31, 32, 94, 95
Influence of the Mind Upon the Body, 30–31

Vesalius, Andreas, 21
Virchow, Rudolf, 25, 26

Waldeyer, Heinrich Wilhelm, 27
Warner, John Harley, 25
Weiner, H., 13
Weiss, Edward, 40
Wernicke, Carl, 27
Wilson, Woodrow, 54
See also Bullitt, William
Wolman, Benjamin, 8, 13

Yelland, Lewis, 171, 172, 173, 182, 184, 185
Young, Allan, 171, 174, 175

Zola, Émile, 63, 93–109
Le roman expérimental, 96
Rougon-Macquart, Les, 63, 99
Thérèse Raquin, 63, 93–109, 117, 195, 197, 198